Sports Medicine for Coaches and Athletes

BASEBALL

Adil E. Shamoo, PhD
*University of Maryland School of Medicine
Baltimore*

Charles E. Silberstein, MD
Sports Medicine Orthopedist

Robert M. Germeroth, PT
*Union Memorial Sports Medicine
Lutherville, Maryland*

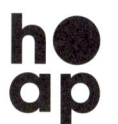

hoap harwood academic publishers
Australia • Canada • France • Germany • India •
Japan • Luxembourg • Malaysia • The Netherlands •
Russia • Singapore • Switzerland

Copyright © 2000 OPA (Overseas Publishers Association) N.V. Published by license under the Harwood Academic Publishers imprint, part of The Gordon and Breach Publishing Group.

All rights reserved.

No part of this book may be reproduced or utilized in any form or by any means, electronic or mechanical, including photocopying and recording, or by any information storage or retrieval system, without permission in writing from the publisher. Printed in Malaysia.

Amsteldijk 166
1st Floor
1079 LH Amsterdam
The Netherlands

British Library Cataloguing in Publication Data

Shamoo, Adil E.
  Sports medicine for coaches and athletes (ISSN 1024-526X)
  Vol. 2 : Baseball
  1. Baseball injuries
  I. Title   II. Silberstein, Charles E.   III. Germeroth, Robert M.
  617.1'027

ISBN   90-5702-611-2

To

Abe, Zach, and *Jessica*
Susan and *Richard*
Jessica, Julie, and *Alexis*

CONTENTS

Introduction to the Series ix
Preface xi
Acknowledgments xiii
About the Authors xv

1 Criteria for Optimal Performance 1
2 Preparations for the Baseball Season 11
3 Management of Baseball Injuries 41
4 Water and Electrolyte Balance for Baseball Players 81
5 Adaptation to Endurance Training 91
6 Nutritional Requirement for Baseball Players 101
7 Drugs and Hormones in Sport 109
8 Gender Difference and Skill Development 115

Further General Reading 121
Glossary 123
Index 133

INTRODUCTION TO THE SERIES

The science of sports medicine and exercise physiology is expanding rapidly. However, this growing body of knowledge is becoming increasingly complex and is not easily accessible to the participants, coaches, athletic trainers, and sports enthusiast most in need of this material. The *Sports Medicine for Coaches and Athletes* series is designed to explain the scientific basis of athletic performance and exercise training by translating complex scientific data into easily understood, practical information and by providing training, nutritional, and injury prevention and treatment guidelines that are specific for individual and team sports and for various groups of exercise participants.

Adil E. Shamoo, PhD

PREFACE

There is a large interest among American youths in playing baseball. There has been advancement in fundamental scientific knowledge relating to sports and exercise physiology, adaptation, and medicine as reflected in the greater number of articles and books on these subjects. However, this information tends to be general and not readily digested by, or directly relevant to, baseball players, coaches, and parents. At times, even physicians, whether pediatricians, internists or orthopedists find it difficult to translate current knowledge into practice. Baseball players and coaches represent highly motivated individuals eager to do their best for the game. Their lack of background knowledge, however, precludes them from utilizing scientific research knowledge accumulated recently in sports medicine for practical use on and off the field. Up-to-date information would help prepare the coach and the athlete for better results in terms of prevention of injury, better training, and adaptation. A proper course of action before, during and after the game and proper rehabilitation, and knowing when to consult a trainer or a physician.

We wrote this monograph because of our strong belief that there was a great need for it; we also wanted to serve the baseball community. Because each coauthor brings his own perspective to the text, this monograph is a unique compilation of ideas, facts, and figures. Adil E. Shamoo has been both playing, coaching, and observing sports events for years; in addition, he taught sports medicine. Charles E. Silberstein is a practicing orthopedist dealing with large numbers of baseball players with various injuries ranging from the benign to the serious. Robert Germeroth is a physical therapist treating baseball player's injuries, rehabilitation, and more importantly, advising them on proper conditioning. This book is written with the players and coaches in mind. The presentation ranges from the very simple to the complex, so that players, coaches, and parents can trace treatment to the scientific logic and reasoning behind the proper practice. It is hoped that the more sophisticated readers will delve into the subject.

To our knowledge, this is the first monograph of its kind. Therefore, we are certain that we may have omitted several aspects of baseball and included others that were not pertinent. In all sincerity, we welcome reader's suggestions, criticisms, and corrections. We plan to revise the text whenever feasible. Please write to Adil E. Shamoo, PhD, Department of Biochemistry and Molecular Biology, University of Maryland School of Medicine, 108 N. Greene Street, Baltimore, Maryland 21201-1503, USA.

ACKNOWLEDGMENTS

Portions of this monograph are taken from our first volume of this series authored by Shamoo, Baugher, and Germeroth either wholly or as an adaptation or modification of certain topics.

ABOUT THE AUTHORS

ADIL E. SHAMOO, PhD
Professor (1979–present) and former chairman (1979–1982) of the Department of Biochemistry and Molecular Biology, University of Maryland School of Medicine in Baltimore, Maryland. Formerly at the University of Rochester School of Medicine, in New York (1973–1979), he also served one year (1972–1973) at the National Institutes of Health. Dr. Shamoo obtained his Ph.D. in Biophysics in 1970 from the City University of New York. His research for the past thirty years has been in the area of biochemistry and biophysics of the skeletal and cardiac muscles. More recently, Dr. Shamoo has been working on dopamine, a brain neurotransmitter. He also taught an elective course to medical students on the "Biochemical Basis of Sports Medicine," 1986–1994. He has contributed to over 200 research papers. In addition, he has edited books and journals, and has chaired numerous international conferences. He is a member of a large number of professional organizations, as well as having held leadership positions, and is a member of the American College of Sports Medicine. Dr. Shamoo has given over 200 lectures worldwide on various topics.

CHARLES E. SILBERSTEIN, MD
Currently in private practice as a pediatric orthopedic surgeon and sports medicine orthopedist of a large sports medicine practice group in Baltimore, Maryland. He is a member of the active staff of The Johns Hopkins Hospital, the Union Memorial Hospital, the Kennedy-Krieger Institute, and the Greater Baltimore Medical Center, and practices at all those institutions.

Dr. Silberstein completed his medical education in 1958 at University of Maryland School of Medicine, Baltimore, Maryland, and a Masters degree in Anatomy in 1964 from Jefferson Medical College. He took his internship at Jefferson Medical College Hospital in Philadelphia, Pennsylvania. He completed his orthopedic residency at Sinai Hospital in Baltimore, Maryland; Jefferson Medical College Hospital; and the State Hospital for Crippled Children in Elizabethtown, Pennsylvania.

In addition, Dr. Silberstein completed a one year Fellowship as a National Institutes of Health Fellow at Jefferson Medical College. Dr. Silberstein is the Director of Sports Medicine at The Children's Hospital and Center for Reconstructive Surgery at its Bennett Institute for Sports Medicine (1978–1985).

Dr. Silberstein has published and lectured widely in the field of sports medicine especially as it relates to hand, wrist, shoulder, and elbow in baseball players. He has been a consultant to the Baltimore Orioles organization since 1966 and was the orthopedic team physician for the Johns Hopkins University from 1972–1992. Dr. Silberstein is an active member of the: American Academy of Orthopedic Surgeons, American Orthopedic Society for Sports Medicine, and the Association of Major League Baseball Physicians of which he was president 1990–1991.

ROBERT M. GERMEROTH, PT, MBA

Currently, site coordinator at Union Memorial Sports Medicine at Lutherville, Maryland. This is one of the largest sports medicine organizations in this geographic area. He received a degree in physical therapy in 1978 from the University of Maryland at Baltimore and a Master's in Business Administration in 1988 from the University of Baltimore. Mr. Germeroth has been a consultant to the Baltimore Orioles and to the Baltimore Thunder; and a large part of his practice deals with baseball injuries. He has made numerous presentations to physicians, athletic trainers, and therapists on the subject of sports medicine and orthopaedics and is a member of the American Physical Therapy Association (APTA), the Sports Medicine Section of the APTA, the Orthopaedic Section of the APTA, and the National Youth Sports Foundation.

Chapter ONE

Criteria for Optimal Performance

Baseball is a major sport for young athletes in the United States, and is also rapidly becoming a major sport for males and females of all ages. Because young athletes go through puberty at different times, there is a great deal of variation among these athletes in terms of size and maturity. These differences pose a challenge to the athletes and to their coaches. The primary characteristics of a young athlete are motivation, physical fitness (i.e., muscle strength, power, endurance, flexibility, proper body composition, and cardiorespiratory endurance), discipline, coachability, skills, ability to be a part of a team, ability to think under stress, and good spatial orientation. Baseball practice sessions should seek to achieve physical conditioning, repetitive training, a proper intensity of training, flexibility, and the awareness that the achievement of proper endurance for the baseball athlete requires at least 4–6 months of training. Also, the coach should be aware that extreme and severe high intensity and high frequency training causes damage to muscle tissues and is counterproductive to the goals of the athlete.

Children and adults have thrown and hit stones with sticks since the beginning of mankind. Stones turn to balls and sticks to bats, but the same hitting of the former with the latter has continued through the centuries. Baseball's most direct ancestors were two British games: cricket, which is divided into innings and supervised by officials, and rounders, a children's stick and ball game brought to New England by the colonists. The current game of baseball was an attempt of Abner Doubleday in 1839 to standardize the numerous variations of ball and bat games being played in America. Since its inception, baseball has been one of the most popular sports in America.

Interest in baseball has continued to grow over the years. It is estimated that more than 2-1/2 million kids under the age of 13 participate in little league baseball every year. This is in part due to the media coverage provided to the sport. During the summer, it is not unusual to find a baseball game on the television or radio. The recent success of the women's softball team at the 1996 Summer Olympics was a catalyst for young people to participate in one of America's favorite past times. There are several senior baseball leagues for those over the age of 50, and in St. Petersberg, Florida a 70 and over league. Colleges are offering more scholarships for men and women to play baseball and softball respectively. Also, with the enormous salaries that professional baseball players are receiving, more boys (and parents of boys) are aspiring to "get to the big leagues."

Baseball is not considered a contact sport, though collisions do occur. The rate of injuries and the severity of injuries in baseball are not as great as in football. It is still not unusual to see various orthopedic problems from playing the sport. These will be discussed in more detail in Chapter 3. Injuries are frequently seen in adult softball leagues, usually because of the poor preparation and condition of the participants.

What then are the factors which contribute to one's performance? Or, perhaps, more importantly, what are the criteria for optimal performance?

PHYSIOLOGICAL AND CHRONOLOGICAL AGE

Those who work with 11 to 16 year old adolescents are aware of the variations in height, weight, strength, speed, coordination and level of maturity which exists in this age group. This is because teenagers, in addition to genetic inheritance of size, are going through puberty which can affect any or all of these factors in various degrees. On the average, the growth spurt occurs around 9–13 (with peak growth rate at about 12) years of age for girls and 12–15 (with peak growth rate at about 14) years of age for boys. Therefore, girls spurt 2 years earlier than boys, which is also reflected in the changes in hormone secretion. Boys usually become slightly taller and heavier than girls after the growth spurt. The young athlete's body is being affected both physically and emotionally because of these hormonal changes. Young people of the same age group who play baseball can and will have a wide variety of skills and abilities. It is, therefore, difficult at times to mold players of various skills and emotions into a cohesive team.

SELECTION OF PLAYERS

There are two types of baseball/softball teams: neighborhood or recreation council teams and travel or select teams. Once in high school, players also have the opportunity to be involved in interscholastic sports by participating in junior varsity or varsity baseball/softball.

Neighborhood teams allow everyone the opportunity to participate. Anyone can register and play for a team with others in their age group. Neighborhood teams normally span in age brackets of two years. There is usually a simple mechanism of evaluating and rating players based on simple skill activities such as throwing, catching, and hitting. Players are then assigned to teams based on their ratings in an attempt to establish some sense of balance between the teams within the league. Selection of players for the travel teams is, like that in high school, based on formal try-outs. The level of skill and play is much better than the neighborhood recreational council games. Despite the selection process, the players still vary a great deal in size and skill level.

CHARACTERISTICS OF A BASEBALL PLAYER

It is not imperative that each individual possess the following characteristics before playing baseball or softball. They should, however, show aptitude and a willingness to acquire these traits.

1) **Motivation**. In baseball/softball, players should show a desire to play the game. The athlete should get enjoyment out of performing the tasks of throwing, catching, and batting without the pressures from adults.

2) **Physical Fitness Traits**. This term can be interpreted in various ways depending on the activity. In the context of baseball, it is the ability to play for two or more hours without physical or mental fatigue, or other symptoms which may interfere with their performance. Each player should have the following physical fitness attributes:
   a) muscle strength and power
   b) flexibility
   c) endurance (especially important for pitchers and catchers)
   d) hand/eye coordination
   e) proper body composition for optimal performance
   f) cardiac respiratory endurance

3) **Discipline**. The player should have the ability to practice and play several times per week. Travel teams often play two or more games in one day on weekends.

4) **Coachability**. The athlete must have the ability to accept instruction, assimilate the information and comply with these instructions.

5) **Ability to learn**. The athlete should have the ability to learn and perform the individual baseball skills of throwing, catching, and batting.

6) **Ability to play in a team sport**. This describes the players ability to work in a cooperative effort with other team members to achieve coordinated play. The player must be willing to sacrifice personal recognition for the sake of the team. The athlete should also be able to associate with other

players for prolonged periods of time and under stressful situations. Each participant should be able to enjoy themselves and their interactions with their teammates.

7) **Ability to think under stress**. Good coaching and practice will train the athlete what to do in various game situations. Though most individuals do not think logically under stressful situations, athletes can learn to think quickly under these conditions.

8) **Spacial orientation**. The athlete must be able to think and visualize an entire playing field and where they need to be at any given moment in various situations. The player should be able to adapt to the spacial orientation within their position and re-position themselves relevant to the ball and other players (teammates or opposing players).

PRACTICE SESSIONS

It is not the intention of the authors to suggest specific exercises or drills. There are numerous sources for these activities and it should be left up to the creativity of the coaching staff to formulate their own style to match the needs of their players. Practices should be enjoyable, as well as educational to achieve maximal benefit and cooperation of each individual participant.

The practice sessions should begin with a light warm-up and stretching program. Skill activity should be performed next in small groups so that each persons' individual needs are addressed. These skills again include batting, throwing, catching, running the bases, etc. Fielding situations can either be incorporated into batting practice or separately, depending on the time allotted for practice. Practices should end with any specific conditioning program the coach may want to include. Conditioning should be left for last as these activities can fatigue the athlete and hinder the skill performance activities.

It is not uncommon for an athlete who plays one sport and then participates in baseball to get sore muscles after the first week or two of practice. This muscle soreness is due to the fact that the muscles are now being used in a different way and frequently utilizing a different set of muscle fibers than in their previous sports. This is referred to as "specificity of training." Thus, the more the athlete participates in baseball/softball, the more their muscles and tendons will adapt to the specific demands placed on them in this sport.

In order to properly *prepare* for the baseball season, players and coaches should observe the following factors:

1) **Physical conditioning**. This involves the athlete's ability to sustain both aerobic and anaerobic activities.

2) **Frequency of training**. This should be two to three times per week for pre-adolescent and early adolescent individuals. It may be three to five times per week for late adolescents and adults.

3) **Intensity of training**. Of primary importance here is the shoulder and arm of the pitchers. A progressive throwing program is outlined in Chapter 2. A slow progressive program is vital to the health and well-being of the pitcher. Baseball is primarily an anaerobic activity. It is still important, however, for baseball players and all athletes to achieve an acceptable level of cardiovascular conditioning. Guidelines for this is also elaborated on in Chapter 2.

4) **Flexibility exercises**. A full range of motion of muscles, joints, tendons, and ligaments is important to maintain proper function of the entire body for baseball. Proper flexibility also decreases the likelihood of certain injuries discussed in Chapter 3. It is not unusual to find inadequate flexibility in the adolescent athlete since the bones are growing at such a rapid rate. This phenomena can be addressed by a properly supervised flexibility program. Since muscle temperature in extremities is slightly lower than core temperature (the trunk), increased circulation of the body into these muscles via calisthenics better prepare the tissue for slow, static stretching routines. A more extensive discussion of this is found in Chapter 2.

5) **Time to peak endurance**. Intense and strenuous training for two to three weeks prior to the season (as is often wit-

nessed in high school sports) will not achieve muscle endurance and, in fact, may be detrimental to the athlete. Adaptation of the cardiorespiratory system and muscle enzymes requires up to six months of training to reach peak endurance capacity. Unfortunately, it only takes two to four weeks without training to lose most endurance parameters (see Chapter 5 on endurance). Therefore, a well-planned, long training period is essential in preparing players for the season. This, again, is particularly true in the case of the pitcher's shoulder. A prime example of this is the training regimen to which most (if not all) major league pitchers adhere. Pitchers usually rest from throwing during the months of October and most of November. In November, they begin a specific strengthening program (see Chapter 2) which they continue into spring training. They begin a progressive throwing program in later November or early December. They continue this progressive throwing program under the watchful eye of the major league coach in January. They continue this right up to spring training, which is usually mid-February. They then continued with a modified (slightly reduced) strengthening program and a progressive throwing program (including games where the pitch count is accurately charted) through spring training. Even with five months (November through March) of preparation, pitchers are still carefully monitored by the trainers and coaches to identify signs of fatigue or injury.

Granted, we are not intending this book for major league players. This scenario is presented only to reinforce the concept of time to peak endurance and adaptation which is so important in the prevention of injuries.

NUTRITIONAL CONSIDERATIONS

A well-devised strength and conditioning program, a sound diet and proper rest are three factors which are required to optimize athletic performance. Of these three factors, the athlete's diet serves as the foundation upon which the other two are based (for details see Chapter 6 on nutrition). Food is the source of fuel for the body to use to build itself, perform athletic endeavors, and repair itself should an injury occur. Only by following basic sound nutritional guidelines can one obtain optimal training effects and, thus, peak performance. There are six nutrients that are essential to the optimal performance of the body. They are:

1) Water

2) Carbohydrates

3) Proteins

4) Fats

5) Vitamins

6) Minerals

These nutrients can all be acquired by routinely partaking in the basic food groups of meats, fruits, vegetables, grains, and dairy products. Water, probably the most important of the nutrients (see Chapter 4 on water and electrolyte balance for baseball players), is essential for the digestion and transporting of the other nutrients to the body. Water also functions to regulate the body's temperature and waste elimination. Carbohydrates are the primary source of energy for the body during intense exercise. Complex carbohydrates (pastas and breads) are better for the body than are the simple carbohydrates (sugars and sweets). Protein is essential for tissue growth, development, and repair. Proteins are important in the formation of hormones, enzymes, and antibodies. They are also another source of energy for the body. Fats provide another source of energy during sustained light to moderate activities. They are also important in the transmission of vitamins A, D, E, and K into the body. Vitamins act as catalysts for utilization of other nutrients, as well as other body functions. Minerals also act as catalysts for such bodily functions as nerve transmission, digestion, and muscle function.

Athletes should consume 60 to 70% carbohydrates, 15 to 20% proteins (approximately 1 gram per kilogram of body weight), and 10 to 15% fat. The exact proportions and quantity should be regulated based on how readily it is used/needed to accommodate the physical demands of training and the athlete's goals of weight control (see the Chapter on nutrition).

PRE-GAME MEALS

Pre-game meals should be planned no less than two to four hours before the game. The closer the meal to game time, the lighter the meal should be. Athletes should also avoid "sweets" just prior to the game or practice to avoid increased insulin secretion (hyperinsulinemia) which, in turn, could result in a lower than normal blood glucose levels (hypoglycemia). Hypoglycemia is felt to be associated with poor performance on the athletic field. Ingestion of glucose during exercise does not result in hyperinsulenemia because of the increased catecholamine secretion (i.e., hormones such as norepinephrine and epinephrine) which suppress insulin secretion. Players should also consume one to two glasses of *cold* water, particularly on hot days, to insure proper hydration. This is particularly important for catchers and pitchers.

During the game, the athlete should drink *cold* water frequently. For every one pound lost during a game, one large glass (400 to 500 ml) of *cold* water should be consumed. It is important *not* to rely on thirst as the impetus for drinking. Pre-adolescent athletes can lose large amounts of fluid quickly and not necessarily be thirsty. Special attention to hydration should take place by those teams playing on artificial turf as the ground temperature is usually higher on such surfaces. Humidity also plays a factor in regulating ones body temperature and, thus, affects the need for water consumption.

HEAVY TRAINING

Fortunately, few baseball coaches resort to very heavy schedules in terms of both the frequency and intensity (e.g., 5 times a week, 4–5 hours per day, with strenuous exercises and high intensity training) of training. If coaches keep the intensity of training high, players may collapse from exhaustion. This type of training is not only detrimental to the individual's well being but also counterproductive to the coach's stated goals. During exercise, muscle protein synthesis is suppressed. Strenuous exercise has been shown to increase the level of muscle enzymes and proteins in the blood, which is indicative of muscle tissue damage. This is because the damaged cells in muscle tissue leak their contents (i.e., enzymes and proteins) to the capillaries and eventually these proteins appear in the blood. This is similar to finding heart muscle enzymes and proteins in the blood after a heart attack. Moreover, severe training could result in the appearance of red blood cells and other blood constituents in urine. This is because of extremely high hydrostatic pressure exerted on kidney blood flow.

FURTHER GENERAL READING

Hong C.Z. and Lien I. (1984). Metabolic Effects of Exhaustive Training of Athletes, Arch. Phys. Med. Rehabil. 65:362–365.

Dohm G.L. et al. (1987). Protein Metabolism During Endurance Exercise, Fed. Proc. 44:348–352.

Kibler, W.B. (1993). Injuries in Adolescent and Preadolescent Baseball Players. Med. Sci. Sports Exerc. 25:1330–1332.

Chapter TWO

Preparations for the Baseball Season

Baseball is a physically demanding sport. To successfully participate in baseball, the athlete must obtain a high level of physical fitness in order to accomplish the anaerobic, sprinting, and skills required for the sport. This chapter offers a brief discussion on the ideal pre-participation physical examination and a physical fitness evaluation. Principles of training requires attention to overload, progressiveness, specificity, frequency, and active rest.

The ultimate source of energy for the body is adenosine triphosphate (ATP). The immediate replenishing source of ATP is phosphocreatine phosphate (PCr). However, ATP and PCr combined will only sustain energy for less than 10 seconds in an exhaustive exercise. Food is processed either through glycolysis (in this process oxygen, O_2, is not utilized; i.e., it is an "anaerobic" process) to yield a quick but yet inefficient source of ATP, or through oxidation (here, O_2 is utilized; i.e., oxidation is an "aerobic" process) which yields a slow and very efficient source of ATP. The anaerobic process produces lactate which contributes to fatigue. Baseball is a mixture of aerobic and anaerobic exercise. Therefore, the athlete should train via a combination of sprint-like exercises, jogging, and running to adapt to both types of exercises.

To be successful at baseball, one must have the strength, power, and coordination along with cardiovascular and muscular endurance to perform these highly skilled tasks. When one considers that in baseball a batter is taking a bat no longer than 42" and no wider than 2-3/4" in diameter, and has less than one second to assess whether or not a 9" in circumference ball weighing five ounces traveling 60' 6" at a speed of 60 to 100 mph is a strike and, therefore, should be swung at, it is no wonder that a person / hitting three of ten balls successfully for a hit is considered an exceptional hitter. It is also little wonder that a fielder must be able to smoothly field this ball, often on a run and then present an accurate throw to a teammate 90+ feet away to be considered a good defensive player. Yes, baseball and softball are highly skilled sports.

A key component to being a successful player is obtaining the physical fitness level necessary to accomplish these anaerobic and skilled movements consistently. Fitness for baseball must address the areas of strength, power, flexibility, muscular endurance, coordination, and cardiovascular capacity.

This chapter will address each of these areas of fitness and their importance in preventing injuries in baseball. Initially, however, a brief discussion on the ideal pre-participation physical examination will be offered, including a physical fitness evaluation.

PRE-PARTICIPATION PHYSICAL EXAMINATION

The athletes pre-participation examination is an integral part of all athletic programs. This evaluation provides a mechanism by which each athlete is thoroughly screened from a physical standpoint, as well as from a fitness standpoint. It is during this time any factor restricting or eliminating an individual from participation is identified. However, such physical examinations are affordable only for college baseball players and beyond. Unfortunately, few high school programs provide such extensive examinations. It is advisable that athletes consult their pediatrician prior to the start of baseball season.

The ideal pre-participation examination is a multi-disciplinary evaluation conducted by a team of specialists ranging from family practitioners, psychiatrist, and internal medicine physicians to orthopedic surgeons. Each physician focuses on their area of specialization, noting those factors which might restrict or disqualify an individual from safely participating in his/her sport. A history of previous medical problems, a general physical examination including an eye examination, and an orthopedic examination are the basic areas a pre-season evaluation should include. Factors such as a history of exercise-induced asthma, high blood pressure, elevated glucose or protein levels, previous head trauma, single paired organs, torn ligaments, or joint pain may warrant further investigation, coaching preparation or disqualification from participation.

PHYSICAL FITNESS EVALUATION

Endurance: The 12-minute run test is a simple and common way of testing cardiovascular endurance. The test has been proven to correlate well with tests that measure maximal oxygen consumption. A high school and college athlete in excellent condition should be able to cover at least 1.75 miles in 12 minutes. For younger athletes, distance should be adjusted proportionally to the age of the athlete. For example, most eight to nine year olds can run a one mile distance in seven to nine minutes. Girls usually run slightly slower in the upper range of the seven to nine minutes.

Strength: An excellent way of screening an individual for strength in through manual muscle testing techniques. This method, when performed under the supervision of a skilled clinician, will point out asymmetries in strength which may warrant further investigation by more sophisticated means such as isokinetic testing. Another common way to obtain a baseline measurement of strength is by using the best score among three trials of a single maximal lift of isotonic weights. It is the authors' opinion that this method should be reserved for those individuals in college or older (if at all) because the risk of injury is high with such activities. Push-ups and pull-ups can be used to measure dynamic strength of the athlete.

Power: The simplest and most common way of obtaining baseline power measurement is through the vertical jump test. In this test, the athlete stands near a wall or measuring device and jumps as high as possible reaching up as they do so. This measurement is compared to the athlete standing and reaching as high as possible without moving or lifting either foot. Isokinetic devices can also be used to measure power, particularly in the upper extremities. Testing on such devices, however, is costly and generally impractical unless rehabilitating in a clinical setting.

Flexibility: Three simple tests can be used to assess the flexibility of the lower extremities. The sit and reach test can indicate tightness of the hamstrings or back. For this test, the individual sits on the floor with knees straight and reaches for the toes. The sacrum (pelvis) should be perpendicular to the floor. If the individuals cannot achieve this position with their pelvis, the hamstrings are too tight. The entire back should form a slow c-curve.

To test for flexibility of calf muscles (plantar flexors), the athlete, sitting with a straight knee, actively dorsiflexors their foot. Using a simple goniometer (measures range of motion), the foot should be able to be pulled back at least 15 degrees. Anything less than this indicates tightness of the calf muscles.

The Thomas test position is an easy and accurate way of assessing the flexibility of hip flexors, quadriceps and iliotibial band. The athlete lies supine with the edge of the table hitting him/her about mid-thigh. One knee is pulled up toward the chest, just enough to flatten the lower back against the table, and the other leg is then allowed to relax and drop to the floor. The back of the thigh of the relaxed leg should rest on the table. If not, tightness of the hip flexors is indicated. The knee should rest at a 90-degree angle. Anything short of this indicates tightness of the quadriceps femoris. Lastly, one should observe if the knee moves away from the mid-line of the body. If so, iliotibial band tightness is indicated.

Flexibility for the shoulder is best evaluated by an individual trained in properly assessing this complex joint. Two simple tests involve the athlete lying supine with their throwing shoulder at the edge of the table. For the test, the examiner lifts the arm enough to be able to stabilize the scapula (shoulder blade) against the ribs. While maintaining this scapular fixation, the arm is lifted to the fully flexed position. The arm should be close to lying flat on the table overhead. The second test involves abducting the upper arm to 90 degrees (out to the side). With the elbow flexed to 90 degrees, the arm is externally rotated allowing the back of the hand to fall down toward the floor. The hand should be able to easily drop below the level of the surface the player is lying on. If either of these tests indicate tightness, a good shoulder stretching program should be followed daily.

Proprioception: Proprioception can be defined simply as the body's sensory awareness of its joint and body position in space. Problems with proprioception can arise from injuries such as ankle sprains. Conversely, if the athlete has had previous injuries to a joint and is not completely rehabilitated, poor proprioception can cause an additional injury. It is, therefore, wise to perform a simple test to assess the proprioception of each athlete. To evaluate proprioception, ask the athlete to balance on one foot. Assess their ability to balance on one foot and compare it to their ability to balance on the other foot. To make the test more difficult, have the athlete close their eyes while balancing on one foot. If the individual has much more difficulty balancing on one foot than the other, further assessment by a health care practitioner (physician, physical therapist, or athletic trainer) and additional rehabilitation may be warranted.

Body composition: Assessing the percentage of body fat a persons possesses is important for two reasons: First, it gives the coach, parents, and trainer (if available) the knowledge of how much weight an athlete can lose safely during the season without losing muscle mass. Well-conditioned male athletes normally possess between 8% and 13% body fat, while well-conditioned female athletes normally possess between 15 and

20% body fat. It is interesting to note that some studies have found that baseball pitchers possess higher percentages of body fat than do the positional players. Secondly, this information can be used to counsel the athlete on the elimination of excess adipose tissue, leading to a healthier lifestyle and enhanced performance levels.

There are numerous ways of evaluating body fat percentages. Underwater weighing is probably the most accurate way; however, it is often the most impractical. The simplest way of measuring the percentage of body fat is through the use of skin fold calibers. In this method, the tester pinches subcutaneous fat between the thumb and index finger, pulling it slightly away from the body. The skin fold calibers are used to measure the millimeters of fat present at a particular spot. Generally, six sites are measured on the body. They include the mid triceps, subscapularis, top of the pelvis, abdominal, upper part of the thigh and mid axillary regions. Measurements are then plugged into any one of several equations (based on age and sex) which, when calculated, provide the evaluator with the percentage of body fat.

PREVENTION THROUGH CONDITIONING

Baseball is primarily a series of anaerobic, ballistic/dynamic activities. Players must possess the explosive power and agility to throw, bat, and maneuver quickly in various directions.

One of the most effective ways of preventing injuries in any sport is to be in top physical condition before and during the season. Therefore, the remainder of this chapter will address the basic concepts needed to properly design a physical fitness program for baseball players. This discussion will not address the topic of skill training activities. Coaches should be well-versed in these skill-related drills also.

ENERGY SOURCE (Figure 2.1)

Required energy varies depending on type of activity, frequency, duration, and intensity. The immediate source of energy for muscle activity within each cell is adenosine

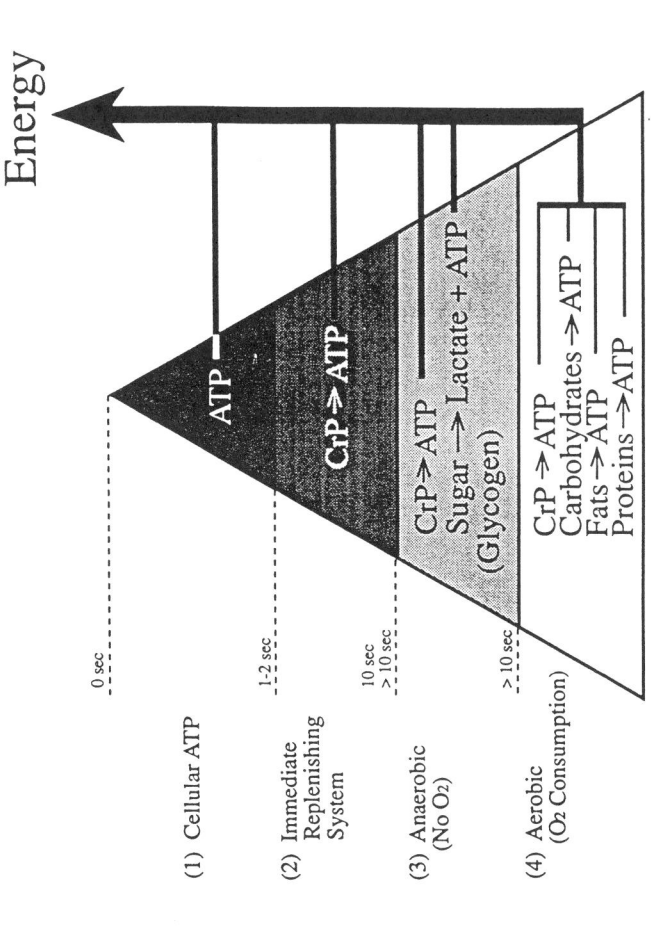

Energy Utilization Pyramid

(1) Cellular ATP — 0 sec — ATP

(2) Immediate Replenishing System — 1-2 sec — CrP → ATP

(3) Anaerobic (No O₂) — 10 sec, > 10 sec — CrP → ATP; Sugar → Lactate + ATP (Glycogen)

(4) Aerobic (O₂ Consumption) — > 10 sec — CrP → ATP; Carbohydrates → ATP; Fats → ATP; Proteins → ATP

Figure 2.1. A hypothetical energy utilization pyramid for baseball players. A baseball player utilizes the needed energy from the available ATP and the quick source of ATP, CrP. This is followed by the next quick source of energy which is supplied by the anaerobic process – this is for when the baseball player engages in bursts of activities. The long range source of energy for baseball players is derived through aerobic processes.

triphosphate (ATP). Muscle action is an organized composite of each cell action. ATP is an intracellular substance which contains three phosphate molecules, and it is through the breakdown of the terminal phosphate that energy is produced. The amount of ATP available in each cell is very small, and only provides sufficient energy to last less than 1–2 seconds in an exhaustive sprint-like exercise. However, the cell attempts to maintain a fairly constant level of ATP, especially during moderate activities. The compound which helps to provide an immediate source of ATP is the molecule phosphocreatine phosphate (PCr). PCr phosphorylates (i.e., adds one phosphate) adenosine diphosphate (ADP) to form ATP. The amount of ATP and PCr combined however, lasts less than about 10 seconds in an exhaustive exercise. The long range source of energy for the cell comes from two main processes that involve utilizing the energy stored in foodstuffs. These two processes are:

(1) **Glycolysis.** ATP is produced anaerobically (without oxygen) from sugar derived from stored muscle glycogen. Glycogen is a polysaccharide (i.e., it consists of many sugars) molecule consisting of hundreds to thousands of glucose molecules linked together. Anaerobic exercise produces lactic acid which can accumulate and have adverse effects on performance. However, the anaerobic process does provide ATP when the body needs it as a quick source of energy (i.e., for sprint-like exercise).

(2) **Oxidation.** ATP is produced aerobically (with oxygen) from carbohydrates, fats, and proteins. The aerobic oxidation process produces 13 times more ATP for the same amount of starting material than ATP which is anaerobically produced by glycolysis. While the aerobic process is slow, it provides long lasting energy for exercises such as jogging and marathon running.

Figure 2.1 gives a hypothetical order of the utilization of energy in baseball playing. Cellular ATP and ATP derived from phosphorylation by PCr are utilized first. Baseball players simultaneously use the anaerobic and the aerobic systems as the situation demands.

A well trained baseball player has an advantage over the untrained person in the utilization of energy. In a later chapter we describe in detail the biochemical changes due to training. However, we will briefly describe the physiological and biochemical advantages of a trained baseball player in utilizing the energy pyramid of Figure 2.1.

In a trained baseball player, the levels of ATP and PCr are higher and thus last about 20–30% longer than in an untrained player. More importantly, the trained baseball player has a greater glycolytic capacity (almost twice as much) as the untrained person. Furthermore, the aerobic system (i.e., enzymes, substrates, etc….) is also more efficiently developed in the trained athlete. The trained athlete can therefore produce ATP faster for the aerobic exercises needed during the game. Above all, the trained baseball player can recover sooner from a bout of exercise because of the increased levels of enzymes, substrates, and capacity to produce ATP.

LACTATE AND FATIGUE

The breakdown of ATP to produce energy results in the production of a hydrogen ion, and thus lowers the cellular pH. This intracellular change in pH eventually lowers the blood's pH. The presence of hydrogen ions is normally a signal for the respiratory system and kidneys to get rid of the excess hydrogen ion. However, under stressful conditions hydrogen ions and/or lactate can accumulate; eventually, the build up of these molecules may contribute to muscle fatigue. Trained athletes physiologically adapt in such a way which allows them to be able to perform adequately in the presence of higher lactate blood levels. Moreover, trained athletes tend to utilize and dissipate lactate better than untrained athletes. Therefore, the specificity of training for a given sport is important in adapting the tissues to those stressful conditions of the given sport in order to stimulate cellular mechanisms of adaptation to those conditions. In general, young athlete have less tolerance to lactate accumulation in the blood than adults athletes.

After an exercise session, it is recommended that an athlete should have a cool-down period consisting of low level activities such as walking or light jogging. This cool-down period helps the blood flow through the capillaries, thus removing lactate from muscles. Rapid removal of lactate from muscles may contribute to the reduction of fatigue. Athletes also may use hot baths or saunas to enhance blood flow to muscles after an exercise session; however, this process is not recommended for players whose muscles are cramped or injured.

FLEXIBILITY EXERCISES

Flexibility can be defined as the range of motion available at a specific joint or with any group of muscles. Though often neglected, stretching exercises are familiar to most athletes. A few basic concepts should be kept in mind when developing a flexibility/stretching program.

First, do not stretch cold muscles. Warm-up calisthenics or jogging should be performed prior to any stretching program to increase core temperature, warm muscles and connective tissue, thus making them more receptive to being elongated. The second concept of flexibility to be considered is the technique to employ when stretching tissues. Ballistic stretching consists of using the momentum of the body to bob in an attempt to elongate the muscle. This type of stretching causes certain muscle receptors to be activated, which, in turn, stimulate the activation of these muscle fibers. The muscle is thus being stimulated to contract while the individual is attempting to stretch the muscle. Though ballistic stretching has been shown to improve flexibility, this type of stretching has the potential to cause musculoskeletal strains. Ballistic stretching is not recommended for these reasons.

Static stretching consists of slowly stretching muscles to a subpainful threshold and maintaining this position for at least five seconds and as long as 20 to 30 seconds. To assure a safe stretch, each stretch should be taken just beyond the point of tightness. Strict form must be adhered to and no movement should be forced, particularly in the shoulder. A thorough stretching program which includes both the upper and lower extremities, as well as the trunk musculature, should be employed prior to practices and game situations.

STRENGTH

Another component of conditioning is strength training. Strength training involves the development of muscular strength, power, and endurance. To understand strength training, one must understand some of the basic physiology of muscle contractions. Aerobic energy systems depend on the availability of oxygen for their production of energy. Carbohydrates, fats, and protein are broken down in the presence of oxygen. This system of energy production allows energy to be supplied to the muscles for several hours.

Another important physiological factor worth noting is that there are two basic types of muscle fibers. Type II fibers (fast twitch fibers) are best adapted for the anaerobic types of activities. Conversely, Type I (slow twitch muscle fibers) are better adapted for aerobic or endurance exercises. Both Type I and Type II muscle fibers can utilize aerobic and anaerobic energy production systems. All muscles are also made up of combinations of both types of fibers. Some individuals have more Type II fibers and are, therefore, more suited for "power" types of activities such as sprinting, batting, throwing, and jumping, while other athletes possess more Type I fibers and, therefore, are more adapted in endurance types of activities. Training programs must be designed to enhance both the fast and slow twitch fibers since each is needed in baseball.

PRINCIPLES IN TRAINING

Building on the foundation of the basic physiologic factors, coaches should consider several principles which must be understood when developing a specific training program for their athletes.

1) **Overload.** The overload principle simply states that in order to build strength, power, endurance, or flexibility, the activity employed must be such that it exceeds in intensity the demands previously or routinely encountered. The overload principle is the foundation for the progressive principle.

2) **Progressive.** The progressive principle states that as an individual begins applying overloads, improvements (i.e., increased strength and endurance) will be experienced. As this improvement is recognized, progressively greater demands (be they heavier weights, more wind sprints, longer sprints, longer throws, etc.) must be imposed or further improvement will not be recognized.

3) **Specificity.** The principle of specificity is particularly important in baseball. The principle states that training should work the muscles involved in a specific sport in the same manner that they will be utilized during the competition. Furthermore, it encourages the development of the primary energy system to be utilized during the competitive activity. A simple example will clarify this principle. It is a fact that baseball involves a great deal of sprinting. If the athlete trains by slowly running three to four miles per day, they will surely enhance their cardiovascular fitness and their aerobic energy system. Baseball, however, primarily involves the anaerobic energy system. The player must be able to sprint around the bases or to catch a fly ball. Therefore, a training/conditioning program which incorporates repeated sprints must be used to improve the strength and muscular endurance necessary to successfully compete in baseball.

4) **Frequency.** Frequency is simply the number of workouts performed in a certain unit of time. To recognize improvement in strength, endurance and skill training must take place on a regular basis. If players do not regularly train, they will lose the strength, endurance, or skill necessary to compete at this demanding sport.

5) **Active rest.** This is often the most overlooked principle when designing a training program. Muscles do not grow during exercise, they are torn down. Hypertrophy (increased size) of muscles and increased strength of muscles and tendons occur during the recuperation period. If constantly stressed without adequate rest, muscles and tendons will eventually break-down and injuries due to overuse will occur.

Active rest consists of low volume and a low to moderate intensity of work which is designed to allow the tissue to sufficiently recuperate. The activity essentially brings extra blood to the tissue in order to flush out the waste products (i.e., lactic acid, etc.), bring additional nutrients, and promote healing to the formerly taxed tissue.

A thorough understanding of these five basic principles will allow a skilled coach the ability to design a comprehensive conditioning program for muscle strength and endurance.

CARDIOVASCULAR ENDURANCE

The most essential component of a well-conditioned athlete is his or her cardiovascular endurance. Cardiovascular endurance can be defined as the ability of the heart, lungs, and blood vessels to efficiently and effectively carry oxygen to the muscles and their connective tissue while simultaneously removing waste products from these same tissues. Approximately 3 milliliters of oxygen per kilogram per minute is the minimum aerobic requirement everyone possesses. The goal of cardiovascular endurance training (aerobic exercises) is to increase the athletes maximum aerobic capacity.

Aerobic training affects the human body in several beneficial ways. The stroke volume (the amount of blood expelled with each pump of the heart muscle) is increased, making the heart a more efficient pump. When the heart rate is increased with exercise, the amount of oxygenated blood is significantly increased. In addition, both blood plasma volumes and the amount of hemoglobin increase with proper training; therefore, the blood can transport more oxygen to the tissue. The receiving tissue also learns to better utilize the increased oxygen that is being supplied. Blood pressure will be lowered. Furthermore, the body becomes more efficient in removing the waste products from the exercise tissue; thus, fatigue does not set in as quickly. Also, recovery time from an injury is decreased.

To successfully improve ones cardiovascular fitness, the rate of exercise must be intense enough to increase the heart rate to 60 to 80% of its maximal rate. To calculate the maximum heart rate of an individual, the following formula is used: 220 minus the age of the person equals maximal heart rate. The intensity must be maintained for 20 to 30 minutes to improve ones aerobic capacity. Furthermore, these workouts (running, bicycling, cross country skiing, swimming, etc.) must be performed three to four times per week at 60 to 80% of the maximal heart rate. Example: A 15 year old baseball player would have to achieve a heart rate between 123 and 164 (220 minus 15 equals 205, 205 times 60% equals 123, 205 times 80% equals 164), maintained for at least 20 to 30 minutes, three times per week to enhance his/her cardiovascular capacity. There are several ways to achieve this high level of intensity as is mentioned above.

STRENGTH AND CONDITIONING PROGRAM

As has been mentioned earlier in this chapter, one of the main reasons to develop a strength and conditioning program is to prevent injuries. This is accomplished by developing good muscle balance between the large shoulder muscles (pectoralis major, deltoid, latissimus dorsi) and the rotator cuff muscles (supraspinatus, infraspinatus, teres minor, subscapularis). Good muscle balance must also exist between the following muscle groups: a) rotator cuff muscles and the scapular stabilizer; b) elbow flexors and extensors; c) pelvic stabilizers and lower extremity muscles. In addition to the balance between the muscle groups, it is also imperative to remain cognizant of the balance between strength and flexibility.

Improved conditioning will also enhance ones recovery time should an injury be experienced. Last, but not least, is the added confidence one will have when they feel better about themselves and their ability to withstand the rigors of training and playing baseball. Below are listed examples of exercises which can be performed:

> Supervision by a qualified professional (strength and conditioning coach, athletic trainer, physical therapist) is strongly recommended, particularly for younger individuals.

INTERVAL TRAINING

The baseball player can benefit from interval training. Interval training consists of workouts with rest intervals varying in ratios from 1:3 to 1:1 (work/rest) depending on the need and the fitness level of the individual. The work period can range from a few seconds to several minutes, and the whole cycle can be repeated 5–20 times. A short, high intensity (sprinting) workout lasting greater than 15 seconds can improve the anaerobic system when interspersed with rest periods of 30 seconds. Interval training to improve aerobic capacity can consist of ratio's of work to rest of 1:1 or 1:1.5. The exercise period can last 60–90 seconds in order to force oxygen consumption followed with a recovery period varying from 60 to 135 seconds.

CIRCUIT TRAINING

Circuit training attempts to economize the time of exercise to improve strength, power, and the cardiorespiratory system. Exercise sessions should combine resistance (lifting weights), repetition, and rest. For example, working periods involving lifting moderate weights can vary from 30–60 seconds with similar rest periods. As many as 15 stations can be included in circuit training.

SPECIFIC PROGRAMS

Running Program
Flexibility Program
Shoulder Strengthening for Pitchers
Upper Body Exercises
Forearm Exercises
Abdominal and Back Exercises
Lower Extremity Program
Medicine Ball Exercises
Progressive Throwing Program – High School and Older
Little League Pitchers

See the following pages for descriptions of these specific programs.

Preparations for the Baseball Season

RUNNING PROGRAM
(4×/week)

- Jog 3–5 minutes to warm-up
- STRETCH THOROUGHLY
- High knee sprints — 120 feet — walk back — 6–8 repetitions
- Back pedal sprints — 100 feet — walk back — 4–6 repetitions
- Cariocas — 100 feet — both directions — 4–6 repetitions
- Shuffle STEPS (side-stepping — don't cross feet over one another like in carioces) — 30 feet — both direction 4 to 6 repetitions
- Sprint 60 yards — walk back — 6–8 repetitions

FLEXIBILITY PROGRAM
(Daily 3–4 repetitions–hold for 20 seconds)

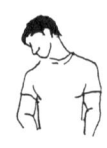

1. NECK ROTATIONS
   Clockwise and counter-clockwise

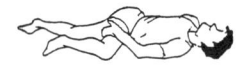

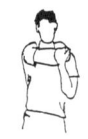

2. PULL ARM CROSSOVER
   Pull arm across body. Both arms

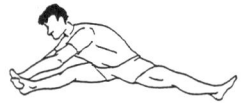

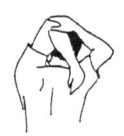

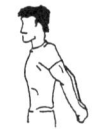

3. PULL ARM BEHIND HEAD

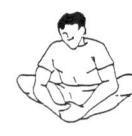

4. BEHIND BACK STRETCH
   Grab hands behind back. Lift arms up keeping elbows straight

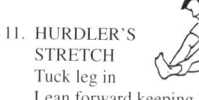

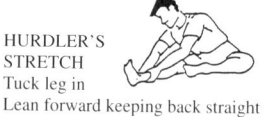

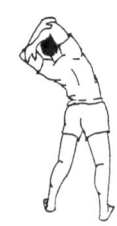

5. UPPER BODY STRETCH
   Same as #3, but also turn body to stretch trunk

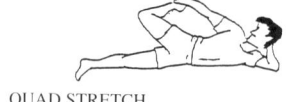

6. TOE TOUCH
   No bouncing Slow steady stretch only

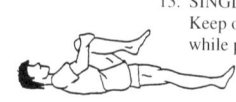

7. LUNGE STRETCH

8. LOW BACK/HIP STRETCH
   Perform slowly

9. STRADDLE STRETCH

10. BUTTERFLY STRETCH
    Soles of feet together pulled towards pelvis Push knees down – lean forward

11. HURDLER'S STRETCH
    Tuck leg in Lean forward keeping back straight

12. QUAD STRETCH
    With pelvis posteriorly tilted, pull leg behind buttocks and hold. Reverse legs

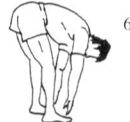

13. SINGLE KNEE-TO-CHEST
    Keep one leg flat on ground while pulling other to chest

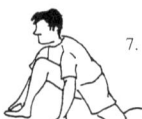

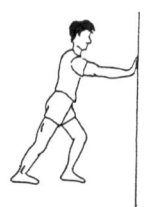

14. WALL LEAN
    While facing wall, place back foot 3–4 feet from wall. Lean pelvis forward while keeping heel of back foot on the floor. Perform with back knee straight and slightly bent. Reverse legs

Preparations for the Baseball Season 29

SHOULDER STRENGTHENING FOR PITCHERS
(off season: 3×/week; in season: 1–2×/week, 3 sets of 15 repetitions)

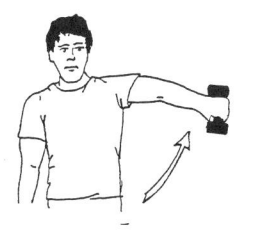

1. **EMPTY CAN (SUPRRASPINATUS)**
   Elbows straight, thumbs down
   Stand in military position with shoulders back
   Lift hand, keeping thumb down, slightly in front of body
   Lift hand to slightly <u>below</u> height of shoulder.
   Do not lift hand above the shoulder

2. **EXTERNAL ROTATION**
   Lying on side with top elbow resting on towel at side
   Raise weight slowly until hand pointing to ceiling, then lower

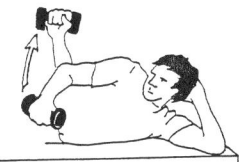

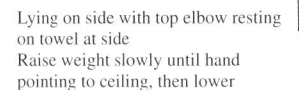

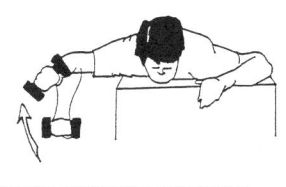

4. **PRONE EXTERNAL ROTATION**
   Lying prone with arm hanging straight down
   Lift elbow such that it is parallel to the floor
   While keeping the elbow bent at 90 degrees, externally rotate the arm as far as possible
   Reverse above sequence and return to the starting position

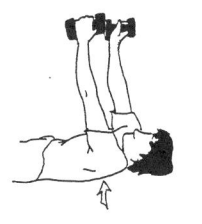

3. **SHOULDER BLADE PRESS UPS**
   Lying on back with arm straight up
   Press weighted hands towards ceiling pushing shoulder blades forward

PITCHER'S SHOULDER PROGRAM (continued)

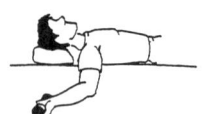

5. **SHOULDER STRETCH**
Place 2–3 lb. weight in hand
With shoulder at 90 degrees and
elbow bent, allow weight to gently
stretch arm down

6. **SHOULDER STRETCH**
Same as #5, but raise arm
another 45 degrees

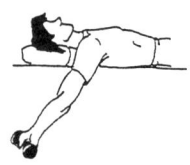

7. **PRONE FLEXION**
While lying on stomach,
lift arms from floor

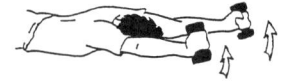

8. **PRONE EXTENSION**
While lying prone, lift weight
up behind back while simultaneously
externally rotating the arm and
pointing the thumb to the ceiling

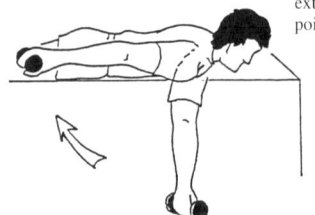

9. **PRONE SIDE RAISE**
Same as #8, but lift arm
straight out to the side

Preparations for the Baseball Season 31

UPPER BODY EXERCISES
(2–3 sets of repetitions each)

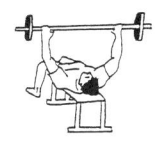

1. BENCH PRESS
   Don't use heavy weights.

2. DUMBBELL ROWS
   Pull elbow up high pinching shoulder blade towards spine.

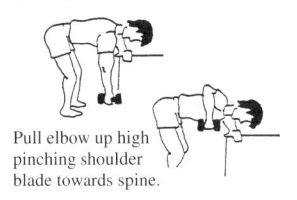

3. LATERAL PULLDOWNS
   Note: Pull the bar in front of head to the chest not behind the neck.

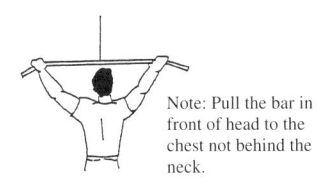

4. SIDE RAISES
   Do <u>not</u> lift the elbow above the shoulders.

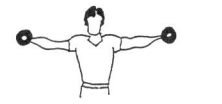

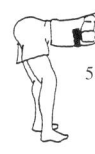

5. REAR SHOULDER RAISES
   Keep arms straight, thumbs pointing up. Raise weight to at least the shoulder level. Lower slowly. This is important.

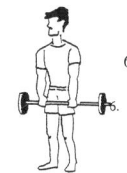

6. SHOULDER SHRUGS
   Hold bar (or dumbbells) and allow shoulders to droop. Raise shoulders up as if trying to touch ears.

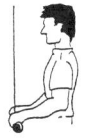

7. TRICEPS PUSHDOWNS
   Slowly push bar down and raise *slowly*

8. TRICEPS EXTENSION
   Keep elbow pointing toward ceiling. Slowly straighten and bend elbows.

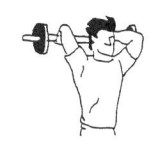

FOREARM EXERCISES
(2 sets of 15 repetitions)

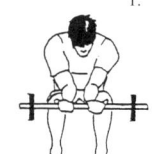

1. **WRIST CURLS**
   Allow wrist to go into full extension and full flexion

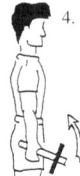

2. **REVERSE CURLS**

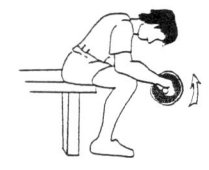

3. **REVERSE BICEPS CURLS**

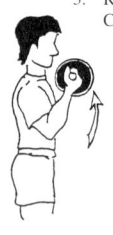

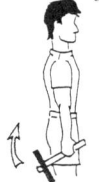

4. **RADIAL DEVIATION**
   Hold dumbbell as far away from the weight as possible.
   Lower and raise bar as far as possible slowly.

5. **ULNAR DEVIATION**
   Same as above, but weight now behind body.

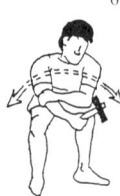

6. **PRONATION/SUPINATION**
   Hold dumbbell as far away from weight as possible
   Rotate forearm as far clockwise and counter-clockwise as possible.

ABDOMINAL AND BACK EXERCISES
(work up to 30 repetitions of exercise, perform each slowly)

1. CRUNCHES

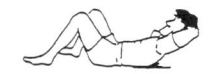

   Lying on back with knees bent and hands behind head
   Lift head and upper back off floor
   Hold for one second and return slowly.

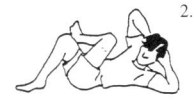

2. ELBOW TO OPPOSITE KNEE
   Lying on back, cross one ankle across opposite knee
   Touch opposite elbow to cross knee

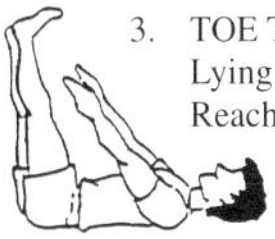

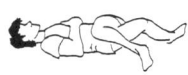

3. TOE TOUCHES
   Lying on back with hips flexed
   Reach up to touch toes

4. ELBOW TO OPPOSITE KNEE BIKE
   Lying on back lift one knee towards opposite elbow
   Alternate right elbow/left knee with left elbow/right knee in a bicycling type motion

5. BACK EXTENSIONS ON BALL
   Place ball under pelvis
   Extend back so it is parallel to floor
   Do not hyperextend the back.

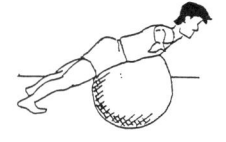

6. PELVIS ROTATION
   Lying on back, the shoulders and upper back are kept on the floor. Cross one leg over the other and rotate the pelvis as far as possible. Reverse legs and repeat.

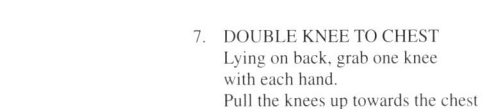

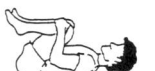

7. DOUBLE KNEE TO CHEST
   Lying on back, grab one knee with each hand.
   Pull the knees up towards the chest
   Hold for 10 seconds.

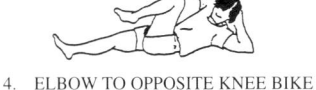

LOWER EXTREMITY PROGRAM

1. SQUATS
   1/2 squat only

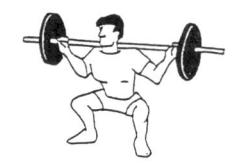

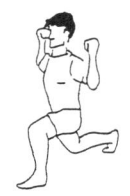

2. LEG PRESS

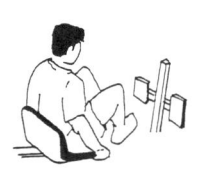

3. STEP-UP
   8–12" step
   Lift and lower body
   with top leg. Do not
   push off the ground with lower leg.

4. LUNGE
   Front leg knees should be behind toes when fully flexed. Torso remains erect.

5. BACK EXTENSION
   Go only to parallel, DO NOT hyperextend back
   Perform slowly

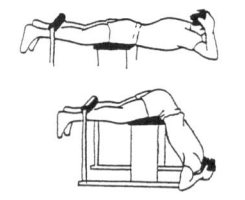

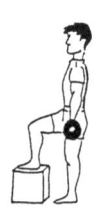

6. TOE RAISES
   Ball of feet elevated on weights or block
   Lift heels high then lower to floor slowly

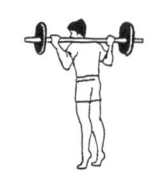

Preparations for the Baseball Season 35

MEDICINE BALL EXERCISES

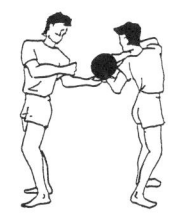

1. FULL TWIST WITH PARTNER
   Stand with feet apart, back to partner about one foot away from one another.
   One partner holds the ball out from the chest.
   While keeping feet stationary, twist torso and pass the ball to partner who is twisting in the opposite direction. Repeat 12 times, then reverse directions.

2. SIDE TO SIDE PASSES
   Stand with feet part.
   Have partner, who is standing in front of you, throw the ball waist high to the outside of one hip.
   You catch the ball twisting to that side.
   Throw the ball back back to your partner.
   The partner will then throw it to the outside of the opposite hip.
   Perform 20 times in each direction.

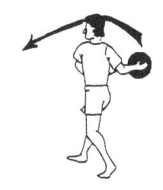

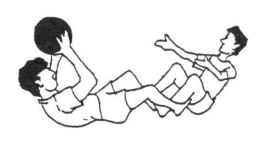

3. PARTNER SIT-UPS
   Face partner with knees bent, feet interlocked and hands overhead.
   The person holding the ball sits up while simultaneously throwing the ball to partner who reclines upon catching the ball.
   Reverse the process.
   Perform 15–20 throws back and forth.

Progressive Throwing Program

Purpose: The progressive throwing program is designed to gradually increase the functional strength, range of motion and condition of the throwing arm, while simultaneously instilling confidence in the athlete and their ability to return to competition. It further emphasizes the importance of energy transfers from the feet through the legs, pelvis, trunk, shoulder, elbow, wrist and hand to the ball.

Goals:
1. To enable the athlete to return to a pain-free competitive throwing level by gradually increasing stress to the throwing arm.
2. To assist in developing a smooth transfer of energy through the *kinetic chain* (feet — legs —

pelvis — trunk — shoulder — elbow — wrist — hand) to the ball.
3. To improve the functional strength and condition of each component of this chain.
4. To increase the endurance of the throwing arm.
5. To educate the athlete on the importance of warm-ups.
6. To minimize the chance of injury.

When Should I Start?: It is advisable for the pitchers to begin conditioning their arm at least 2–3 months before the start of the season. Position players should begin throwing a minimum of 6 weeks before practice begins.

General Guidelines:
1. Properly warm-up the entire body by jogging or performing simple calisthenics (Goals: Light sweat)
2. Thoroughly stretch all muscle groups beginning with the legs and progressing through the pelvis, trunk, arms and ending with the shoulder (8–10 minutes).
3. Begin throwing under the guidance of a knowledgeable health care profession (physician, therapist, trainer) and/or coach. Perform each step for two consecutive days, rest for one day, then progress to next step.
4. *NEVER* progress to the next step if pain was encountered during the previous one. *STOP!*
5. Follow the progression rigidly. DO NOT skip your prescribed steps. If you increase the intensity too fast, you will increase your risk of injury and may delay your return to competition.
6. Perform your strengthening exercises of high repetitions (15–20 reps) and low resistance (5–6 lbs) on the same day(s) that you throw after throwing unless otherwise instructed.
7. Stretch after performing the throwing *and* strengthening exercises.
8. Ice the rehabilitated area (front and back) for 15–20 minutes after exercising.
9. Use the off day for flexibility exercises and ice, if necessary.
10. EXPECT SOME SORENESS, but *not* pain.

HIGH SCHOOL AND OLDER (Pitchers and Fielders)

A. 45 FT. PHASE -
   Step 1: Warm-up throws
   Throw 6–8 minutes
   Step 2: Warm-up throws
   Throw 8–10 minutes

B. 6O FT. PHASE -
   Step 3: Warm-up throws
   Throw 6–8 minutes
   Step 4: Warm-up throws
   Throw 8–10 minutes

C. 9O FT. PHASE -
   Step 5: Warm-up throws
   Throw 6–8 minutes
   Step 6: Warm-up throws
   Throw 8–10 minutes

D. 12O FT. PHASE -
   Step 7: Warm-up throws
   Throw 6–8 minutes
   Step 8: Warm-up throws
   Throw 8–10 minutes (Crow-hop)

Steps 9 & 10 are optional for pitchers *only*.

E. 150 FT. PHASE (Pitchers' mechanics must not change)
   Step 9: Warm-up throws
   Throw 6–8 minutes (Crow-hop)
   Step 10: Warm-up throws
   Throw 8–10 minutes (Crow-hop)

HIGH SCHOOL AND OLDER

PITCHER'S PROGRESSION (Following completion of step 8)
P1 Warm-up throwing
    Fast balls 1/2 spd (6–8 min.)
    Long toss 90–120 ft (3–5 min.)
P2 Warm-up throwing
    Fast balls 1/2 spd (8–10 min.)
    Long toss 90–120 ft (3–5 min.)

P4 Warm-up throwing
    Fast balls 3/4 spd (6–8 min)
    Long toss 90–120 ft (3–5 min.)
P5 Warm-up throwing
    Fast balls 3/4 spd (8–10 min.)
    Long toss 90–120 ft (3–5 min.)
P6 Warm-up throwing
    Fast balls full spd (4–6 min.)
    Rest (4–6 min.)
    Fast balls full spd (4–6 min.)
    Long toss
P7 Warm-up throwing
    Fast balls full spd (3–5 min.)
    Rest (3–5 min.)
    Breaking pitches 3/4 spd (3–5 min.)
    Rest (3–5 min.)
    Fast balls full spd (3–5 min.)
    Long toss (2–3 min.)
P8 Warm-up throwing
    Fast balls full spd (3–5 min.)
    Rest (3–5 min.)
    Breaking pitches 3/4 spd (3–5 min.)
    Rest (3–5 min.)
    Breaking pitches 3/4 spd (3–5 min.)
    Rest (3–5 min.)
    Fast balls full spd (3–5 min.)
    Long toss (2–3 min.)
P9 Warm-up throwing
    Fast balls full spd (3–5 min.)
    Rest (3–5 min.)
    Breaking pitches 3/4 spd (3–5 min.)
    Rest (3–5 min.)
    Breaking pitches full spd (3–5 min.)
    Rest (3–5 min.)
    Fast balls full spd (3–5 min.)
P10 Warm-up throwing
    Fast balls full spd (3–5 min.)
    Rest (3–5 min.)
    Breaking pitches full spd (3–5 min.)
    Rest (3–5 min.)

Preparations for the Baseball Season

       Breaking pitches full spd (3–5 min.)
       Rest (3–5 min.)
       Fast balls full spd (3–5 min.)
P11   Batting Practice
P12   Game

FIELDER'S PROGRESSION (Following completion of step 10)

F1   180 Ft (Crow-hop)
      Warm-up throwing
      Throwing 6–8 min.
F2   180 Ft. (Crow-hop)
      Warm-up throwing
      Throwing 8–10 min.
F3   210 Ft. (Crow-hop)
      Warm-up throwing
      Throwing 6–8 min.
      Rest 5–6 mm.
      Throw 6–8 min.
F4   240 Ft. (Crow-hop)
      Warm-up throwing
      Throwing 6–8 min.
      Rest 5–6 min.
      Throw 6–8 min.

LITTLE LEAGUE PITCHERS

A. 30 FT. PHASE
     Step 1:   Warm-up throwing 20–25 throws
     Step 2:   Warm-up throwing 25–35 throws
     Step 3:   Warm-up throwing 35–50 throws

B. 45 FT. PHASE
     Step 4:   Warm-up throwing 25–30 throws
     Step 5:   Warm-up throwing 30–45 throws

C. 6O FT. PHASE
     Step 6:   Warm-up throwing 25–30 throws
     Step 7:   Warm-up throwing 30–45 throws

D. 90 FT. PHASE (*Athlete should not strain to throw this distance)
   Step 8: Warm-up throwing 25–30 throws
   Step 9: Warm-up throwing 30–45 throws
   Step 10: Warm-up throwing 45–60 throws

E. Pitching Mound
   Start at 1/2 speed for 20–25 throws progressing slowly to 3/4 speed and then full speed working up to 3 sets of 20–25 throws with a 3–5 minute rest between sets.

Chapter THREE

Management of Baseball Injuries

Baseball related injures require management both at the time of, and for some time after, the occurrence of an injury. Acute and immediate management is aimed at preventing further damage to tissues until definitive healing and rehabilitation can take place. The removal of the athlete from the field of play (if deemed appropriate by the initial evaluation) immediately following any injury allows the player to rest and gives the manager/coach and the player adequate time to thoroughly evaluate the injury. The key to the immediate management of injuries in most cases is RICE (rest, ice, compression, and elevation). RICE is an effective and prudent treatment for most baseball injuries, and involves little if any risk. Injuries that last several days and are associated with pain without remission or with increasing pain should be referred to a physician who has the capability and training necessary to properly evaluate and treat sports related injuries. Most of the baseball injuries are chronic in nature due to overuse or microtrauma and they more often affect the shoulder and elbow. Chronic injuries require careful evaluation followed by proper rehabilitation. The prevention of chronic injuries requires adequate pre-season preparation and avoidance of overuse.

MANAGEMENT OF BASEBALL INJURIES

Unlike football, soccer, tennis, and running, the injuries which occur in baseball are unique because the preponderance occur in the upper extremity, in particular the shoulder and elbow. Rather than these injuries occurring acutely, most are the results of overuse and the cumulative effects of "wear and tear." Many of the injuries which appear to occur acutely in the shoulder and elbow are in actuality sudden aches and pains that result from some pre-existing microtrauma to a tendon, ligament, or muscle. Whereas tennis players may practice their strokes several hours a day, pitchers workouts are limited to just a few minutes or less than 50–75 pitches. So why then do we see fewer shoulder and elbow problems in the younger (less than 35 years old) tennis players as opposed to those who throw baseballs? Perhaps this is related to the mass and weight of a baseball in a player's hand as opposed to the racquet being an extension of the upper extremity. The cocking motion to serve a tennis ball is not unlike the cocking motion in throwing a baseball.

Baseball players will also sustain injuries of the lower extremities (Figure 3.1). Hamstring and quadriceps muscle strains and tears occur most frequently when running the bases. These can occur as a result of concentric contraction of these muscles as when taking the first few running steps out of the batter's box or as the result of eccentric contraction — in particular in the hamstrings — during deceleration at each base. Knee and ankle injuries most often occur during sliding into bases or in collisions at each base. The use of a "breakaway" bases in amateur softball leagues has been found to

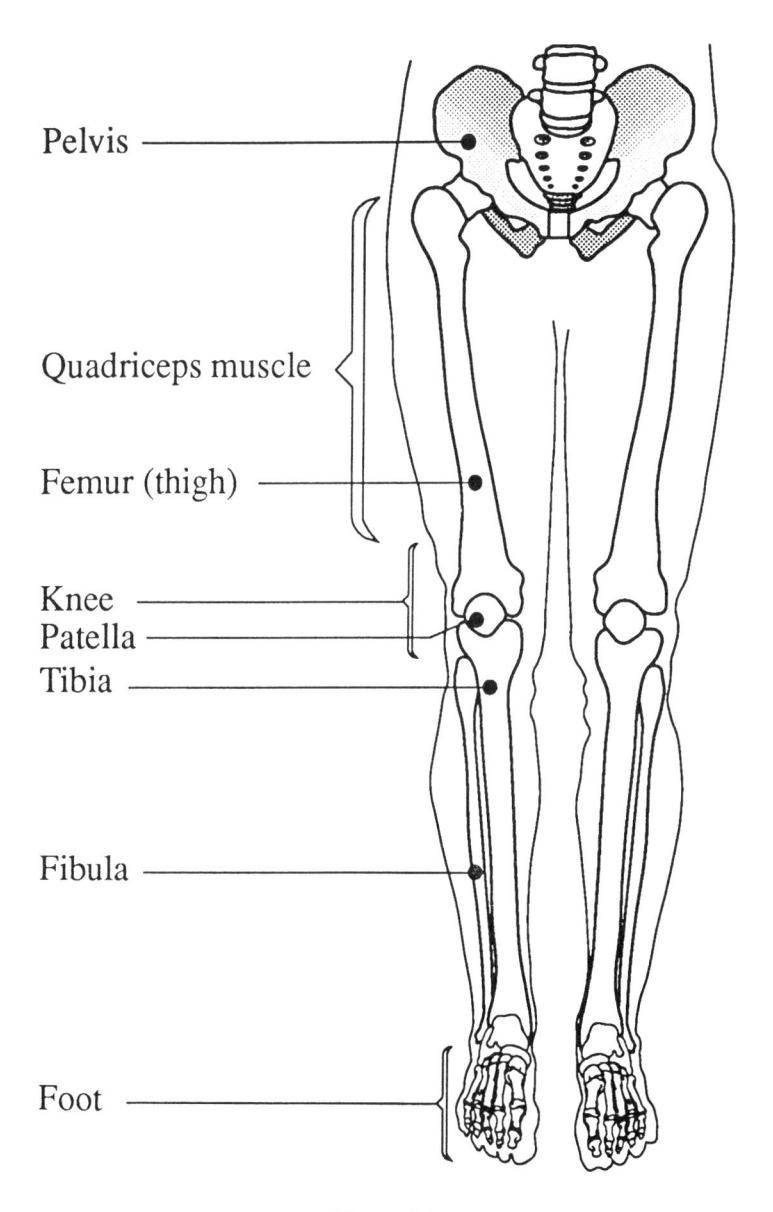

Figure 3.1.

have a profound effect on decreasing the incidence of ankle injuries.

Back injuries are uncommon in amateur baseball unless pre-existing pathology exists, such as the developmental abnormality of spondylolisthesis.

Diving to make a catch can lead to shoulder separations (acromioclavicular — AC — joint) and tears of the triangular fibrocartilage (TFCC) in the wrist. Diving head first into a base can be associated with shoulder subluxations ("I felt something pop").

Studies on body fat composition in baseball players have shown that at the professional level, infielders tend to have the lowest levels and catchers and pitchers tend to be higher in body fat. One study was done with respect to mortality in professional baseball players and showed that infielders tended to live longer than those at other positions.

Facial injuries — orbital and maxillary fractures can be rather severe and of serious consequences if facial flaps are not worn on batting helmets.

WHAT TO DO WHEN AN INJURY OCCURS ON THE FIELD (see Figure 3.2)

Since most youth baseball teams will not have a physician or a trainer present, the manager/coach, players, and parents must be prepared to recognize the severity of any injury that occurs during the play. If in doubt, the injury must be treated as though it were serious. When an injury does occur, do not immediately move the injured player until you ascertain from your own observations and that of the player the type and severity of the injury. If the player cannot get up on his own, then he should not be moved. The coach should always err on the side of safety. If the player has difficulty with vital signs (breathing, pupil size, pulse, sensation, speech, consciousness), then an ambulance should be called. In extreme situations CPR may have to be given (by a qualified person) if there is severe difficulty in breathing. In rare instances, there have been isolated cases of sudden death from cardiac contusion due to a pitched ball striking the chest of the batter. Most

Management of Baseball Injuries

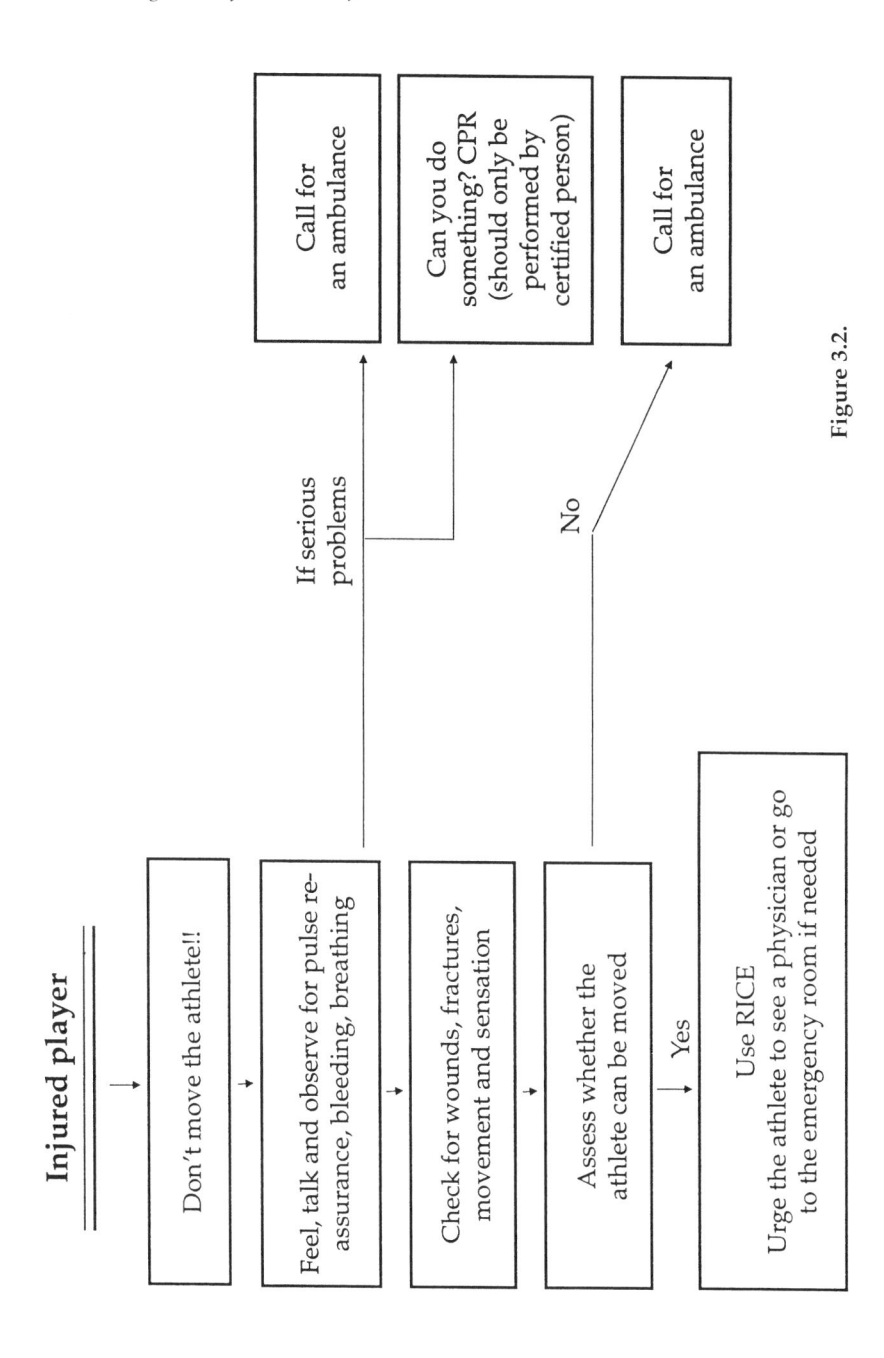

Injured player

→ Don't move the athlete!!

→ Feel, talk and observe for pulse re-assurance, bleeding, breathing — *If serious problems* → Call for an ambulance → Can you do something? CPR (should only be performed by certified person)

→ Check for wounds, fractures, movement and sensation

→ Assess whether the athlete can be moved — **No** → Call for an ambulance

Yes ↓

Use RICE

Urge the athlete to see a physician or go to the emergency room if needed

Figure 3.2.

of these injuries can frequently be treated by simply applying first aid techniques on the field; however, more serious injuries, such as broken bones, require hospital or physician assistance.

Most common injuries in sports are due to overuse. Any physical activity causes changes in the tissue that requires readjustment and a healing period. Overuse of muscles is due to either too much exercise or too frequent exercise within a period of time without a sufficient rest period for recovery. Cross training, combining the use of different muscles on different days, is valuable in providing rest periods. If the pattern of overuse continues, it can lead to rupture and damage or failure of the muscle tissues. Common examples of injuries due to overuse include sites of shoulder and elbow. The three types of tissue injures are listed below:

Contusions: This is a blow to soft tissue such as muscles and skin and involves capillary and cellular damage.

Strains: This is an injury to the matrix of a muscle or a tendon (a tendon is the connective tissue which joins the muscle to the bone). This is usually a pulling or traction type injury.

Sprains: This is a partial or complete tear of a ligament. A ligament is a supporting tissue that holds the bones of a joint together and allows motion only in the appropriate plane. A good example is the medial collateral ligament of the knee.

All athletic injuries are caused by either macro-trauma or micro-trauma. Macro-trauma is relatively easy to understand. It occurs when an overload of force is applied to an anatomical structure. Since the force can not be resisted, the anatomical structure fails mechanically. Micro-trauma occurs subtly. Micro-trauma is caused by repeated small insults and injuries to an anatomical structure. No one small application of force is sufficient to create overload. The small forces occur with enough frequency over a relatively short period of time to compromise a biological mechanical structure. That structure is unable to repair itself rapidly enough to prevent ultimate failure. The most common site in baseball of this type of trauma occurs in the shoulder and elbow (little league elbow).

RICE

RICE is an acronym used by trainers and other sports medicine personnel for the initial treatment of most injuries. It stands for rest ice, compression, and elevation. If there is any question regarding the severity of an injury, this is a reasonable and prudent manner in which to begin treatment.

Rest

Rest may be immediate or delayed, partial or complete. Certainly, in its most basic form rest implies taking an injured player out of the game or practice situation and giving him/her adequate time to recover. In overuse injuries rest may be relative, such as a decreased activity level rather than the complete cessation of activity. Rest for injured body parts may include splints, casts, and nonweight bearing with crutches.

Ice

Lowering the temperature of a traumatized area to approximately 3° to 4°C (or about 37–39 Fahrenheit (F)) is important to reduce further injury to tissue. This is called cryotherapy. Cryotherapy, an ancient technique which was practiced as far back the Grecian Empire, involves the use of cooling to reduce trauma to an injured area and to initiate rehabilitation. In any injury, tissue is damaged and the injured region undergoes a healing process. Secondary to the injury, there are two detrimental occurrences that can cause further tissue damage, and these are enzyme release and hypoxia (reduced oxygen). Hypoxia can cause further cell death which can lead to additional damage. The application of ice to the injured area yields the following benefits:

1. Reduces regional metabolism and oxygen utilization. Cryotherapy results in a greater chance for tissue survival.

2. Reduces degradation of healthy tissue by the enzymes released from the damaged region.

3. Induces vasoconstriction to the damaged area and thus reduces further damage and swelling. Prolonged

cryotherapy may allow vasodilation of the area; thus, the intermittent use of ice for 20 to 30 minutes at a time may be more effective than ice alone.

4. Delays inflammation or the actual release of inflammatory enzymes.
5. Has an analgesic affect that often allows proper mobility and prevents a painful reflex arch.

Therefore, the early application of ice after an injury is very helpful in the overall treatment of the injury. Cryotherapy should be applied for 15 to 20 minutes several times a day for the first 48 hours following an injury. Heat is *not* recommended in the first two days after an injury. However, after two days contrast treatment, that is alternating heating and cooling, may be used (see attached contrast schedule in Figure 3.3). The use of wet ice is probably the most effective

CONTRAST BATH

```
Hot water temperature:   102 degrees
Cold water temperature:  50 to 55 degrees

*   START IN THE COLD WATER AND END IN THE COLD WATER
```

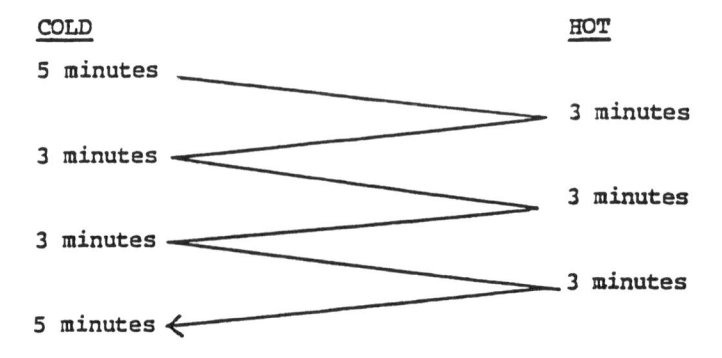

COLD	HOT
5 minutes	
	3 minutes
3 minutes	
	3 minutes
3 minutes	
	3 minutes
5 minutes	

Figure 3.3.

and quickest way to reduce tissue temperature. Wet ice may be more effective than cold packs because it can provide a greater surface area for contact with the injury.

Compression

Compression may be used as a part of splinting or simply to control edema (accumulation of fluids) and swelling. It is important to remember that compression is quite different from strangulation which can cause circulatory compromise. In other words, a modest compression dressing that does not cut off the circulation will help control pain and edema and will help to splint the injured area. The most common method of compression is an elastic wrap, but caution must be exercised not to make the wrap too tight.

Elevation

Elevation is also a method of edema control and helps to ensure rest. Elevation means that the injured body part is elevated in reference to the right side of the heart. The right side of the heart defines the pressure of venous return of the circulatory system or the drainage from an involved limb. Therefore, to effectively elevate a lower extremity, the patient must be in a recumbent position.

It is difficult to decide which injuries are minor and will improve on their own, and which injuries require referral to a consulting physician. Obviously, the extremes are easy to identify as any manager/coach or player can recognize a minor ankle sprain which one can "walk off" and recover from in a matter of minutes. Conversely, a displaced fracture requiring a trip to an emergency room is also easy to identify. The problem arises when there are injuries that effect play on a subtle basis; in these instances, the method of treatment may not be obvious. In these cases the authors recommend referral to an orthopaedic surgeon certified by the American Academy of Orthopaedic Surgeons. One may choose a surgeon who has a special interest and expertise in sports medicine. As a matter of ethics and courtesy, and even financial necessity, depending upon the changes we see in medical practice, it is often appropriate to use a primary care physician to initiate a referral. Many players, both young and old, will more readily consult their manager/coach regarding an injury than parents, family, or physician. This may place a burden and responsibility on coaches to attend various coaching seminars on first aid and injury identification.

The remainder of this section will discuss selected injuries that are common to baseball. It is obviously impossible to cover all injuries but an attempt will be made to highlight the injuries that most commonly occur on the baseball field.

LOWER EXTREMITY INJURIES (see Figure 3.1)

Injuries to lower extremities in baseball are infrequent but nevertheless they do occur.

1. **Blisters.** The most common injury is the simple blister. In an ideal situation, all baseball players would come to practice with shoes that were well broken in; in addition, the player would have developed appropriate calluses on their feet. Unfortunately, this is not always the case. Frequently, in the beginning of the season players will have new, poorly broken in, or poorly fitted shoes. In addition, often at the beginning of the season, players are not in good physical condition. All of this can lead to blister formation on prominent areas in the foot. A blister is an irritation of the superficial layer of skin until it loses attachment to the underlying layer; this space is frequently filled with fluid. Blisters should be kept clean. Often an extra pair of socks or adequate padding and a petroleum jelly gauze over a blister will enable the player to continue to participate. The fluid in a blister is generally sterile and routine puncturing of a blister is not advocated. However, at times drainage under sterile conditions or spontaneous drainage or rupture will decompress the blister and allow a more rapid return to play.

2. **Turf Toe.** This is a sprain or injury to the supporting structures around the toe joint from hypertension or repeated hyperextension. In the foot itself, a common injury is a sprain of the 1st metatarsal phalangeal joint, frequently called turf toe (see Figure 3.4). This can occur either from an acute

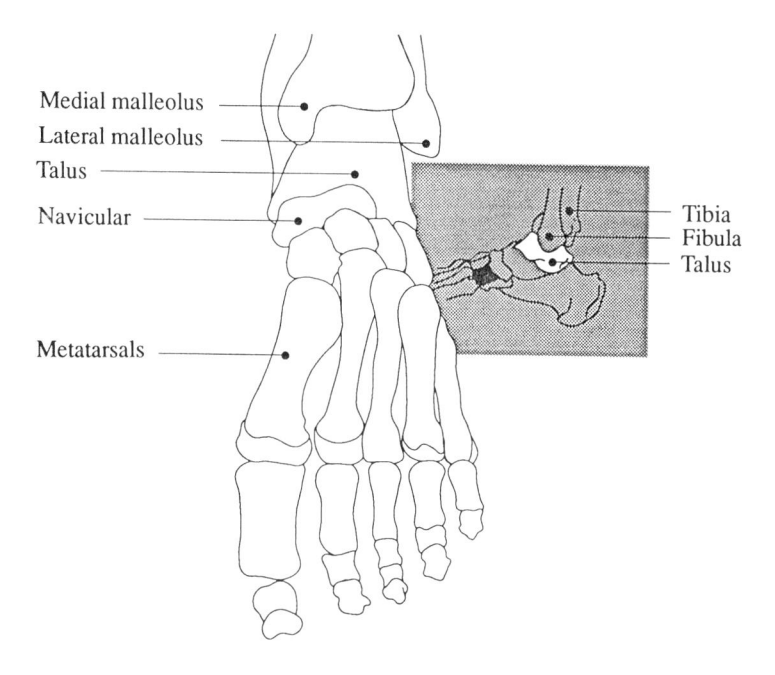

Figure 3.4.

episode, or can be the result of a repetitive injury. It is more frequently seen when playing on a hard surface such as artificial turf or an indoor field. On these surfaces less rigid shoes are used which also contributes to the problem. It is impossible to adequately immobilize this joint for complete healing and still allow continued play; therefore, only rest will cure this injury. Frequently, players with turf toe continue to play; however, the injury will be a nagging problem throughout the season resolving only when the toe is allowed to rest and heal.

3. **Foot.** Twisting injuries to the foot can result in a sprain of the tarsal, metatarsal, or intermetatarsal joints. This can lead to localized swelling, persistent pain, point tenderness, and difficulty pushing off the foot. If a player has pain in the mid foot area, the foot should be evaluated early with adequate x-rays. If one misses an acute injury and does not treat it until it becomes chronic, it may preclude conservative or non-surgical management. Surgery for a chronically stretched ligament

may require arthrodesis (immobilizing the joint) which will result in loss of foot motion. A fracture or stress fracture of the navicular may also be present with pain in the mid-foot area (see below).

a. **Flat Foot/Plantar Fasciitis** (see Figure 3.5). A foot with a relatively flat arch may be predisposed to injury. The most common injury in this situation is plantar fasciitis. This condition results in pain along the plantar fascia which runs along the plantar or under surface of the foot. This tissue acts as a "truss" to support the normal arch of the foot. If this area is abnormally stretched either acutely or through repetitive loading and unloading of the foot, it may lead to pain which is most often felt at the insertion of the fascia into the heel. The common heel spur is really due to irritation of the plantar fascia as it inserts into the heel itself.

With this type of injury pain along the arch and a stiffness of the foot is felt most acutely upon first arising. The pain decreases a little as the foot is limbered and loosened by walking, but is felt again with increased activity, as the entire complex of symptoms is aggravated by increased activity. Appropriate treatment involves the use of anti-inflammatories, ice, and arch supports or taping. Cases which do not respond to this conservative management scheme need to be referred for expert evaluation to make sure that there is no abnormality in the bony structure of the foot which may play a part in causing this pain.

Individuals with high arches also have a very tight plantar fascia and are predisposed to plantar fasciitis.

b. **Sever's Apophysitis.** This is a condition due to relative overuse or micro-trauma seen at the insertion of the Achilles tendon into the heel. There is a growth center or aphophysis at the insertion of the tendon that may be aggravated by activity. This area is also prone to inflammation and irritation because of a potential weak point where the tendon inserts near the cartilaginous center of the growth plate. Injuries in this area are best treated symptomatically and should disappear when the player reaches skeletal maturity. Icing, anti-inflammatories and, frequently, a small heel lift will often relieve symptoms. If the heel lift does not provide relief, one can consider prescription orthotics for the treatment of this condition.

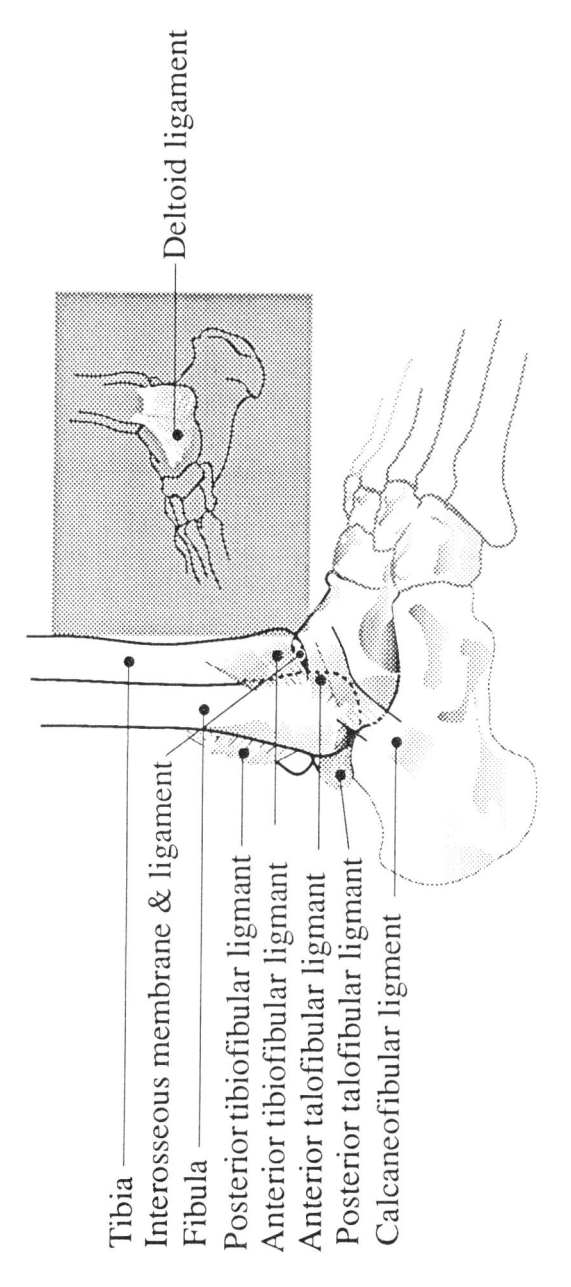

Figure 3.5.

c. **Stress Fractures.** Stress fractures are common in the foot. They occur whenever stress or activity induced remodeling of the bone occurs so rapidly that the deossification (the antonym of ossification; ossification is defined as bone formation) stage outstrips the repair stage. Examples for conditions that could cause stress fracture are running indoors on hard surface and outdoors when there is a prolong drought that causes the ground to become hard. This leads to a negative turnover of hard bony tissue. Tenderness and inability to bear weight are the signs and symptoms that contribute to the diagnosis of a stress fracture. Pain that persists, even after cessation of activity, such as in the evening or morning after playing is an important symptom. The most common area of occurrence for stress fractures is the 2nd metatarsal; however, any metatarsal may be affected. Persistent pain in any area in the foot is a mandate for referral and x-ray evaluation. If an x-ray does not show specific changes, a bone scan may be necessary to make the appropriate diagnosis. Almost all stress fractures can be successfully treated with simple restriction of activity. That is, limitation of running, jumping, and walking great distances. This type of injury usually does not require splinting or nonweight bearing treatment. Treated in this manner stress fractures almost always heal, but if a stress fracture is ignored it is not inconceivable that the patient may go on to fracture through the stress fracture converting it to a displaced fracture that needs more aggressive treatment.

There are several stress fractures which require greater vigilance and more aggressive treatment. One of these is a stress fracture at the base of the 5th metatarsal. A stress fracture in this area must be watched carefully as these have a potential for nonunion and can require operative intervention. Another area of concern is the navicular. This is the bone in the mid-foot area where the 1st and 2nd metatarsals join the mid-foot. Fractures of this bone are best treated with nonweight bearing and immobilization. Unrecognized fractures of the navicular may lead to arthritis, and can require a fusion for successful treatment. While this may decrease pain, it will significantly limit motion in the foot. If there is reproducible point tenderness to palpation in any bone in the foot, one must consider referral for evaluation of a stress fracture.

d. **Sprain.** A sprain is a medical term which describes a torn ligament. The most common ankle injury seen in all sports, including baseball, is the lateral ankle sprain. The ankle joint is a mixture of ligaments and tendons with inherent bony stability. The lateral ligaments are the weaker ligaments in this joint compared to the medial ligaments. There are three lateral ligaments that attach the fibula, or outside bone of the leg, to the talus and calcaneous of the foot. These ligaments prevent the ankle from rolling over or inverting. A sprain to these ligaments occurs when a player lands on the outside of his foot in such a manner as to twist his body over it or roll the foot underneath. The degree of the tear can vary. Significant tears which do not cause limping can be successfully treated with icing and strapping, and one might continue play while a minor sprain heals. More significant sprains will need support of the ankle through taping, strapping, or braces, and some of these treatments will allow resumption of play in these orthotic devices. Significant sprains require x-ray evaluation because there is no other way to insure that one does not have a fracture. It is important to remember that younger players have an epiphysis (growth plate) at the tip of the fibula which is just as likely to be injured as the ligament. In fact, it is relatively common for the epiphysis to be injured or even avulsed or pulled off because the junction of the epiphysis to the bone itself is weaker than the ligament. If the epiphyseal injury is nondisplaced, this can be treated with immobilization just as with a severe sprain, but the injury should be recognized and properly diagnosed. The degree of swelling and the degree of functional impairment are the determining factors in deciding whether or not to refer the player to a physician for evaluation. Treatment may require a period of immobilization in order to allow the sprain to heal; once the sprain has healed, protective devices such as splints or braces and taping should be utilized in order to allow an early return to play. It is important to make sure that normal mobility and strength is restored to the ankle prior to full return to unrestricted activity. A referral to a certified trainer or physical therapist may expedite rehabilitation.

Medial ankle sprains or deltoid ligament sprains are rarer than those just discussed above, and can be treated in a similar manner. Again, in cases of persistent swelling and soreness it is important to get an x-ray to avoid missing a fracture, particularly of a growth center. The mechanism that causes a sprain can also cause an avulsion fracture off the base of the 5th metatarsal. This is a smaller piece of bone and more proximal than the stress related fracture. These fractures will most often heal with rest and immobilization.

LEG

Clearly, the most common injuries to the leg are contusions and hematomas from contact with another player. It is important to treat these with extra pads; in particular, a foam doughnut can be made in order to protect or take pressure off a sore area.

a. **Compartment Syndrome.** The muscles in the lower leg, particularly those in the anterior compartment, are invested with a thick supporting tissue called fascia. This forms a rigid sleeve around the muscle and a contusion, fracture, or even extreme overuse can cause the muscle to swell inside of this confining tissue. Swelling can create pressure to such a degree that it can cut off the relatively low pressure capillary inflow which the muscle depends upon for its nourishment. Compartment syndrome occurs when the pressure leads to ischemia or a loss of blood supply to the muscle. This type of injury constitutes a surgical emergency and requires release of this tight structure in order to allow the muscle to survive. The hallmark of this diagnosis is severe pain in the muscle itself. Lack of a pulse distal to the involved area has also been described as a part of this syndrome, but frequently a pulse may be readily apparent while the muscle above is still ischemic. Paresthesias, "funny feelings," or numbness are common, but anyone with severe pain should be evaluated on an emergency basis, because the only reliable way to exclude acute compartment syndrome is with direct measurements of the tissue pressure.

b. **Stress Fracture.** A very common area for stress fractures is the tibia. It is often difficult to differentiate a stress fracture from shin splints; however, stress fractures seem to have a more focused or localized area of direct tenderness to palpation and require a period of rest. The diagnosis is usually made by x-rays, but occasionally the x-rays are normal. If several x-rays are normal and pain is persistent, it is worthwhile to obtain a bone scan to make sure that there is not a stress fracture that is not yet apparent. Again, the treatment for stress fractures is avoidance of impact activity. This type of injury does not prevent one from bearing weight, but running should be prohibited. Consequently, sports activities may be prohibited until the fracture is healed, usually over a 6 to 8 week period. It is important to remember, however, that non-weight bearing activity and fitness activities such as biking and swimming can be used to maintain fitness during the healing period. Weight training may be included in the rehabilitation and is not contra-indicated by stress fractures.

c. **Shin Splints.** Shin splints are most frequently caused by overtraining. They are probably best described as a reactive peritendinitis or an inflammation of the insertion of a muscle into the bone. There are some anatomic conditions which predispose players to the development of shin splints; in these cases, the incidence of shin splints can be decreased with appropriate foot wear and orthotics. However, the essential factor in the prevention of shin splints is a gradual increase in training coupled with adequate flexibility. Sometimes it is extremely difficult to differentiate between shin splints and a stress fracture without an x-ray or a bone scan. The severity and frequency of the pain lead one to make a clinical judgement as to the appropriate time for obtaining these studies.

There are, as mentioned, certain conditions that have a causal effect with regard to shin splints. One condition is overtraining and another is an anatomic predisposition. When players stay fit in a year round conditioning program overtraining is less of a problem. An athlete should gradually, but not precipitously increase the amount of running. Predisposition of an anatomic nature usually involve mechanical problems with the lower foot. This can include an extremely rigid and highly arched foot or a very flexible flat foot. Either of these conditions prevents the proper damping of forces throughout the lower extremity when the foot and lower limb are exposed to the constant pounding and impact seen with running. Properly fitted orthotics or shoe inserts are often very helpful in this situation, particularly when coupled with the appropriate use of modalities such as ice.

KNEE (see Figure 3.6)

The knee is frequently injured in many sports and is often a source of pain and disability. When dealing with young athletes it is important to remember that hip pain may be referred to in the knee much in the way that someone suffering from a heart attack feels pain radiating down his arm. If a young player is complaining of knee pain particularly with the lack of localized findings about the knee, consideration should be given to evaluation of the player's hip as well. When dealing with the knee, it is helpful to think of general categories of injuries and problems. The first would be knee stability, the second the extensor mechanism and its various afflictions, and the third would be internal derangements of the knee. Internal derangement are problems that exclude the extensor mechanism or stability but can cause significant knee malfunction.

a. **Stability.** The knee as a joint operates within certain degrees of freedom. It is allowed to bend and extend in some planes but is restricted in others. It is allowed to rotate in a limited manner but is tethered by the ligaments to prevent it from excess motion in certain directions. The ligaments are composed of thickened connective tissue and are attached to either side of the knee joint. The most commonly injured ligament is the medial collateral ligament which is a broad flat ligament that runs down from the medial femoral condyle to the tibia. Thus, it runs down the inside of the knee and crosses the joint acting like a leather strap or hinge. This ligament allows the knee to bend and extend but stops the lower leg from moving away from the body or to the side. The most common injury is when someone is struck from the outer aspect of the knee and the knee bends inward. This stretches or damages the medial collateral ligament. Most of these injuries or sprains require a period of immobilization to allow a damaged ligament to heal. Milder injuries may be treated with mobility and a hinged brace.

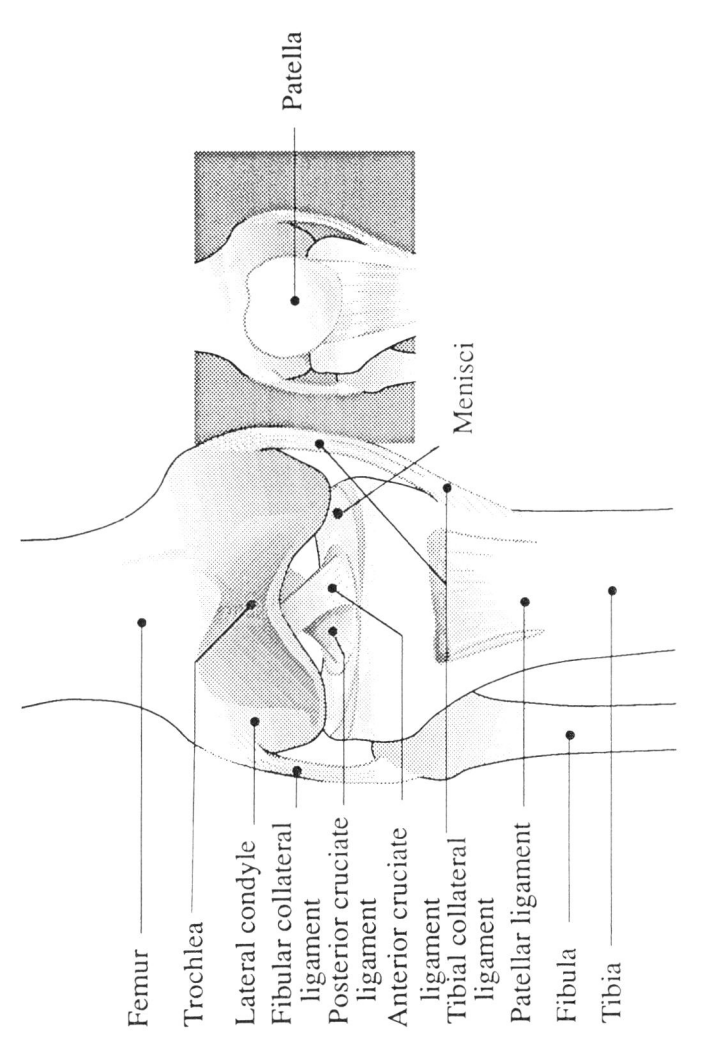

Figure 3.6.

Femur
Trochlea
Lateral condyle
Fibular collateral ligament
Posterior cruciate ligament
Anterior cruciate ligament
Tibial collateral ligament
Patellar ligament
Fibula
Tibia
Patella
Menisci

In younger players there are growth centers or epiphyses about the knee that may be weaker than the ligament. Unlike a ligament injury, in young players the growth center may be pulled apart or opened up; thus, a subtle widening of this epiphysis may be seen on x-ray. This indicates a fracture through the growth center rather than a ligamentous injury. In other cases ligaments may pull off or avulse a small piece of bone. All significant injuries to the knee should be evaluated with an x-ray.

The next common ligament injury of importance involves the tear of the anterior cruciate ligament (ACL). The anterior cruciate is a ligament that is inside the knee, and it runs from the tibia, or lower bone, of the knee to the femur, or upper bone. It runs obliquely across the center of the knee from the anterior medial or inside portion of the tibia to the posterior superior and lateral or outside aspect of the femur. This ligament is injured with twisting or with a sudden deceleration or stop on the knee accompanied with a twist. It can also be injured by a severe force applied to the outer aspect of the knee which first damages the medial collateral; when this ligament is completely torn, anterior cruciate ligament may also be damaged. An injury to this ligament results in significant knee swelling and there is disability whenever the player or patient attempts to change directions quickly. In most patients damage to this ligament will prevent successful participation in baseball because a baseball player must obviously be able to run, turn, and slide. Injuries to this major ligament to the knee must be referred to the appropriately trained person for treatment, as this ligament can not be repaired without surgery. 80% of acute ACL ruptures will be associated with a "POP".

b. **Extensor Mechanism.** The extensor mechanism consists of the quadriceps muscles, or the anterior thigh muscles, with their tendon inserting into the patella. The patella, or kneecap, and the patellar tendon, which is the tendon beneath the kneecap, joins this mechanism to the tibia. Thus, when the quadriceps muscles contract they extend or straighten the knee. This is the strong muscle of the anterior thigh that propels the body forward when the leg is planted on the ground. Injuries to the muscles themselves will be discussed below under thigh injuries. The kneecap may be damaged in many ways; for example, a direct blow may cause a contusion.

Sometimes the kneecap will slip or be forced off to the side of the knee thus dislocating or subluxing it from its position. Subluxation is a partial dislocation of the kneecap which is quickly pulled back into place. Milder forms of subluxation that occur over time may be treated effectively with an exercise program and perhaps knee alignment braces. These braces are made of soft neoprene or rubber with a hole cut out for the kneecap and a pad on the side to prevent the kneecap from sliding laterally. These braces are quite light and do not preclude player participation at a high level. The more severe forms of this condition will become evident and may require surgical treatment. In this type of knee injury surgery should not be entertained as a solution until a course of nonoperative management has been attempted and found to fail. One exception is an acute injury with a one time forceful dislocation of the kneecap. This is a true traumatic event and may necessitate immediate repair. Fractures of the kneecap may require surgery, but this depends on the nature of the fracture seen on the x-ray.

c. **Tendon.** Below the kneecap is the patellar ligament (or tendon). This tendon attaches the kneecap to the tibia. This is the last link through which the force is transmitted from the muscle to the lower leg. This tendon is often stressed by repetitive use and pounding on the leg as seen in running sports, particularly on hard surfaces. Frequently, tendinitis may occur from relative overuse. Counter force braces or padding, ice, and, again, a gradual increase in the level of activity are the best ways to prevent and treat these types of injury.

Osgood Schlatters disease is a special type of irritation of the patellar tendon. This occurs in an athlete with an open epiphysis or growth center in the knee. The patellar tendon attaches directly to this area and is a potentially weak spot. Repeated stress on the patella tendon may cause injury and fragmentation to the growth center. This condition is usually reversible and is treated with a counter force brace, with limited running but continuation of play.

d. **Internal Derangement.** The term internal derangement of the knee encompasses many different areas. The three most common areas include plica syndrome, meniscal tears and, particularly in adolescence, osteochondritis dissecans.

(1) **Plica Syndrome.** A plica is a fold of synovial tissue that stretches across the inside of the knee. It is often a normal finding but can become symptomatic if this tissue becomes inflamed, scarred and hardened. When this occurs the tissue can rub or irritate the knee when the knee goes through a course of flexion and extension. It may result in pain and swelling in the knee. Symptoms include frequent pain on the inside aspect of the knee over the femur; at times, the plica can actually be felt through the skin. Conservative or early treatment consists of the proper use of ice and anti-inflammatories, and can even include a course of supervised physical therapy. When this pain becomes intractable to the point that it interferes with activity and can not be controlled by conservative management, arthroscopy and excision of the plica by surgical methods may be indicated.

(2) **Meniscus.** The meniscus is a fibrocartilaginous tissue that can act as a washer or spacer and shock absorber inside the knee. There are two of these structures in each knee forming an inner and outer or medial and lateral meniscus. They are semicircular in shape and embrace the condyles of the femur. The meniscus is attached to the joint and can be damaged in twisting type injuries. If a meniscus is completely torn, surgical excision or repair may be required. The signs of a meniscal injury include recurrent swelling of the knee, pain, and tenderness, particularly along the joint line. At times, prior to considering arthroscopic or surgical intervention, special imaging procedures such as MRI (Magnetic Resonance Imaging) may be helpful in making the diagnosis. MRI is an expensive test, and should be used only when necessary; at times, it is more appropriate to proceed to arthroscopic evaluation without an MRI.

(3) **Osteochondritis Dissecans.** Largely seen in adolescence, this condition occurs when a portion of the joints' surface, or more precisely, the bone directly under the cartilage surface of the joint may temporarily lose its blood supply. This can result in fragmentation of the cartilaginous surface of the bone. Often, rest of the knee or cast immobilization will allow this injury to heal. Occasionally, operative treatment is

required, particularly if there are free fragments in the knee. The signs of this injury are swelling and pain. There is often tenderness to direct palpation or touch, particularly when the knee is flexed by the examiner. This diagnosis can frequently be made with plain x-rays, but at times MRI may be required to confirm the diagnosis.

In summary, the warning signs for significant knee injuries are pain, swelling, locking, or instability. These are injuries that should be fully evaluated prior to resumption of play in order to prevent further injury.

THIGH

Thigh muscles consist of two groups of large muscles — quadriceps (anterior) and hamstrings (posterior). Sprains and tears of these thigh muscles are in baseball usually due to deceleration as when attempting to slow down.

Strains and contusions of the thigh muscles are the main injuries occurring in the thigh. Strain implies a tearing of the muscle fibers when a sudden acute overload is applied to them. This is most commonly seen in the quadriceps muscle. The quadriceps are the muscles that extend the knee. When someone is sprinting, they may overload the muscle and tear the fibers. This, as with most muscle injuries, should be treated with rest in order to facilitate healing. These muscle injuries almost never require surgery and can be treated in a conservative manner. These muscle injuries can be graded into I (mild), II (medium), and Ill (severe). This classification of I to Ill is old but still useful so that treatment can be optimized and more importantly, lends an appreciation to the time it takes each grade to heal and recover. Grade II and Ill tears are notoriously under-treated. A major mistake made is an early return to play when the player feels better but the muscle, while having partially healed, has not healed well enough to allow vigorous activity. The early return to activity could result in frequent re-injuries and prolonged disability. As with any other injury acute injuries are treated with ice.

A Grade I tear will usually heal within 10 days and is treated with rest, ice, and compression for 24 to 48 hours and then gradual stretching, contrast baths (i.e. hot and cold) after two days and graduated running and agility drills. Grade II tears require more fibroblastic proliferation (special types of cells) for healing and are rested for 10–14 days and usually take 4–6 weeks to heal. These are treated by the same protocol as in Grade I but strengthening exercises and running in a pool can begin at approximately three weeks. Grade Ill tears require a longer period of maturation for the fibroblast proliferation and can take 12–16 weeks to heal and the protocol for treatment is the same as in Grade II.

The adductor muscles are also commonly injured in this manner. This is frequently referred to as a groin pull or strain. The muscles that are tender or damaged are the ones that pull the leg into the mid-line or adduct. Appropriate stretching and warm-up will prevent a lot of these injuries from occurring or recurring. In the acute instance, a certain amount of rest is required. Taping and strapping has been found to be helpful in symptomatic relief, but one must be mindful of the fact that this is a physiological injury, and must be given time to heal.

Often in a younger patient an injury to the entire quadriceps mechanism will result in an avulsion of bone from the pelvis. This can occur because the muscle inserts into a relatively weak area on the bone and the muscle contraction and muscle tensile strength is stronger than that of its insertion into the bone. A similar injury can occur with the hamstring muscles as well. Thus, if there is any severe pain or swelling, particularly at the bony insertion of the muscle, an x-ray of the pelvis may be helpful in making a diagnosis. These bony avulsions seldom require surgery or re-attachment, but do indicate the severity of the injury and are helpful in determining the amount of rest necessary.

Contusions of the thigh muscles are seen when a hard object such as a foot or a ball strikes the anterior thigh area. This results in the well known "charlie horse." Obviously, these are difficult to prevent as they are a common mishap which occurs rarely during a play. Once these injuries do occur it is critical to ice them immediately to prevent bleeding and residual stiffness and soreness. Compressive wraps, non-weight bearing and rest until the muscle can be stretched out and function in a normal contractual manner again are the major treatments for this injury.

HIP

The most common injuries to the hip are mentioned above (that is, bony injuries), but there is another form of bony injury that is also quite painful. This is the "hip pointer." This type of injury refers to an avulsion or an injury through a contusion to the abdominal muscles off the superior edge of the pelvis or hip. This can be quite painful and difficult to control and may require rest for a period of time. Ice and anti-inflammatories as well as rest are the appropriate treatments for this type of injury.

One potentially disastrous problem seen in the hip is the slipped capital femoral epiphysis. In a growing child with open epiphyses even the simple forces of daily activity can cause the growth center of the end of the femur or the round head that inserts in the hip socket to slip. This is truly an emergency situation in that neglect or improper early care can lead to severe arthritic changes in the hip which are difficult to salvage by any means. Thus, if a patient has any limping or loss of motion around the hip, it is important to realize that this particular condition can occur with very little trauma.

UPPER EXTREMITY INJURIES (see Figures 3.7 and 3.8)

Upper extremity injuries especially the shoulder and elbow are more common in baseball than other sports. They are usually caused by repetitive overuse.

In order to best diagnose a shoulder or elbow problem in a throwing arm, the player should be able to provide the physician with answers to the following key questions:

1. Starter or reliever
2. Arm slot — over-the top, 3/4, side arm
3. Pitch selection — types of pitches commonly used — fastball, curve-ball, etc.

4. During which phase of throwing — early or late cocking, acceleration, release, follow-through. By knowing which muscles and ligaments are being stressed during the

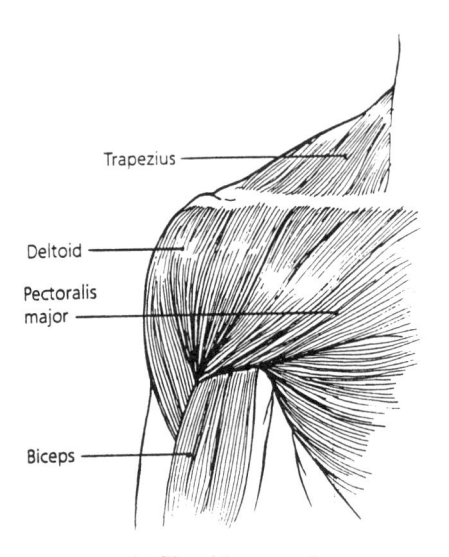

A. Shoulder muscles.

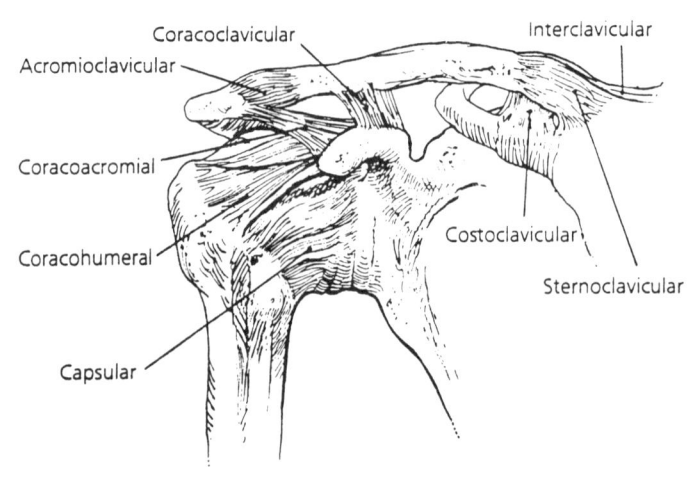

B. Ligaments of the shoulder.

C. Glenohumeral joint.

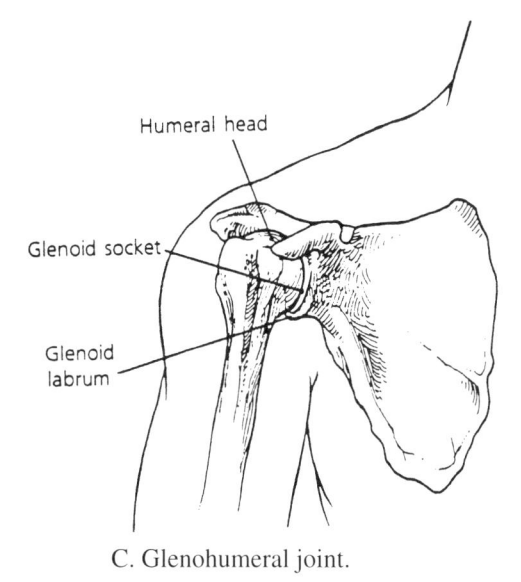

Figure 3.7. The major components of the shoulder.

throwing cycle, the examiner can then key on these during the examination.

5. Number of innings pitched.
6. Loss of velocity and/or location — this can occur as a result of injury but not necessarily associated with any other complaints.

The biceps and triceps are primarily active at the elbow and not at the shoulder.

The physician will relate the symptoms to underlying anatomy and pathology. For example, anterior pain may indicate biceps tendon, glenohumeral instability, or torn anterior labrum. Lateral pain may indicate rotator cuff, and posterior pain may indicate rotator cuff, glenohumeral instability, or torn posterior labrum.

Tightness may indicate problems in capsular region or rotator cuff tendinitis vs. tear.

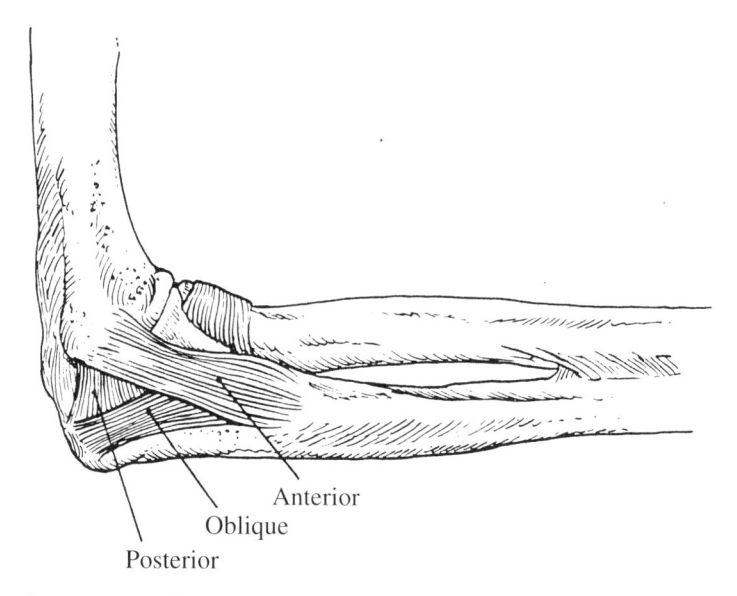

Components of the Medial Collateral Ligament

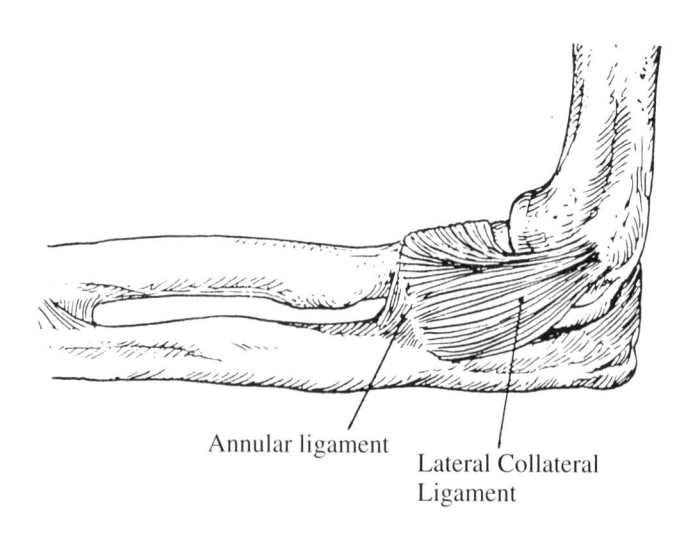

Figure 3.8. Elbow.

Clicking and popping may indicate any one or a combination of the following:

Instability
Torn labrum
Rotator cuff tears
Loose bodies

With instability there is excessive movement of the humeral head (ball) within the glenoid fossa (socket) due to laxity and stretching of the joint capsule. This may be due to inherent increased elasticity of the capsular tissue associated with "looseness" of other joints or it may be due to wear of the labrum-front or back- and stretching of the inferior genohumeral ligaments due to repetitive throwing. As the humeral head slips over the edge of the socket it may produce a click or a pop. A piece of torn labrum may get caught or trapped between the humeral head and glenoid during the act of throwing. A fragment or edge of torn rotator cuff may get rubbed between the acromion and the humeral head or the greater tuberosity causing catching. Finally a loose fragment of bone that has broken off and floats freely within the joint can cause a sensation of popping or catching.

"Deadarm" may indicate any one of the following conditions:

Instability
Circulatory problems
Fatigue

Instability will cause a asynchrony of movement between the head of the humerus, the glenoid fossa and the surrounding muscles. This lack of synchronous motion can effect nerves (suprascapular and/or axillary) in the area and the excessive relaxation of the tissues can cause a sensation of what the player refers to as a "deadarm". With the arm in the cocking position-excessive external rotation with abduction — the axillary artery or the posterior humeral circumflex artery may be compressed and there may be a decrease of blood flow causing a sensation of "deadarm". This same mechanism has been shown to cause clotting in the axillary artery with small clots breaking off and going to the small vessels of the hand

and fingers causing a loss of circulation. Obviously fatigue from overuse can cause a sensation of "deadarm".

Diagnosis: In order to establish an accurate diagnosis, the examiner must have a basic understanding of the biomechanics of pitching and know which areas of the throwing arm are associated with specific pathological conditions. Therefore, as in any aspect of medicine, first obtain an accurate history. Sir William Osler, the first Professor of Medicine at the Johns Hopkins University, School of Medicine, has said that if you listen to the patient he or she will tell you what's wrong with them. Important questions to be asked are: Has there been a loss of velocity? Has there been a loss of location? Do you every have a sensation of deadarm? Do you ever feel a sensation of clicking or popping in your shoulder or elbow? For pitchers with elbow complaints it's important to note whether or not they have had any previous shoulder symptoms which may have caused them to drop their arm more to the side when throwing, which results in more strain on the inner aspect of the elbow.

The examination of the athlete should begin with the examiner standing behind the player and inspecting the shoulder girdle for any obvious atrophy or wasting of muscles around the shoulder-girdle on the dominant side. A not uncommon finding is atrophy of the infraspinatus muscle on the lower half of the scapula (shoulder blade). This is usually due to entrapment of the suprascapular nerve. Then have the athlete raise his or her arms forward (both simultaneously) as far as they can and then out to the side as far as they can. Watch to see if both motions are smooth and symmetrical. With rotator cuff weakness or damage, once the arm gets above 90 degrees, the individual may unconsciously perform a hunching motion and substitute the trapezious muscle. Then observe from the front. Look for any obvious gap between the edge of the acromion and the humeral head (sulcus sign). Pull down on both arms simultaneously and see if a gap appears or if each side shows the same degree of gap. This is a tipoff that there might be some multidirectional instability in the shoulder. To check for stability see the preceeding section 4.

As a result of obtaining an accurate history and then performing a comprehensive physical examination the trainer, therapist, or physician who has obtained all of this information should have a pretty good idea as to what the most likely diagnosis is. At this point it may then be necessary to obtain some form of imaging study, such as plain radiographs, MRI, or CT arthrogram so as to verify your diagnosis. Plain radiographs (x-rays) are useful in evaluating the bony labrum and, in the skeletally immature, evaluating the status of the growth plate. In the older individual they are helpful in evaluating the contour of the acromion, which may tip one off as to the chances of significant impingment of the rotator cuff. MRIs show all of the soft tissues in great detail. However they can be too sensitive. There have been 2 separate studies which have shown a 30% incidence in rotator cuff tears in asymptomatic young men. CT arthrograms are useful for detecting glenoid labrum tears. There are a limited number of centers that have become adept at using Ultrasound (realtime) to evaluate rotator cuff tears. In the final analysis, when treatment has been unsuccessful, the ideal way to evaluate the joint is with an arthroscope (a surgical procedure).

Other conditions that occur in the shoulder are tendinitis of the biceps tendon or strains of this tendon and labral tears. Biceps tendon problems frequently occur as a result of the thrower "opening up" too soon, that is turning the landing foot out too far which results in the pelvis rotating too far and the pitching arm lagging behind. This usually responds quickly to rest, icing, and nonsteroidal anti-inflammatory drugs. Obviously the best treatment is to improve the thrower's mechanics. Labral tears are frequently associated with instability problems in the shoulder. On examination a palpable clunk may be felt when the humeral head is pistoned back and forth while the patient lays supine. Another test is to have the athlete sit with his or her hands on the hips an apply a loading pressure to the elbow, up through the arm to the shoulder. Pain with this maneuver may indicate a tear of the labrum where the biceps tendon attaches.

1. **Rhythm.** Have player flex both shoulders simultaneously and watch for scapular winging as arms are raised and then lowered. Do the same for shoulder abduction. This is a check for scapulohumeral rhythm. With rotator cuff pathology once the arm is above 90 degrees of abduction, there may be a com-

pensatory hunching of the shoulder due to trapezius compensation for cuff weakness.

2. **Range of Motion (R.O.M.).** To check range of motion, the key range tested, when standing, is external rotation versus internal rotation. Most athletes will have excessive external and less internal rotation when compared to the opposite side. To check functional external rotation, abduct the shoulder 90 degrees and then externally rotate as far as possible. Normally, this should be at least 30 degrees beyond neutral or 120 degrees. To test internal rotation, have the hand reach behind the back with the thumb touching the spine. On the non-throwing arm, the thumb should reach at least 3–4 spinous processes more proximal than the throwing arm.

Then check the R.O.M. with the patient lying supine with the head flat on the table. Stabilize the scapula to the rib cage and while holding the scapula, bring the arm into overhead elevation or flexion. This should be at least 120 degrees. Then carry the arm across the body, again with the scapula stabilized on the rib cage. The elbow should come at least 3 inches beyond the midline of the body.

Tightness or limitation in the range of motion are predisposing factors which can lead to muscle-tendon strains and tears.

3. **Strength.** Manual muscle testing is carried out by having the player use isolated movements to resist the pressure of the examiner's hands. Several static and dynamic tests should be administered in order to isolate and diagnose the injury.

4. **Stability.** This refers to both the dynamic as well as the static stability of the glenohumeral joint. Dynamic stability is provided by the muscular control of shoulder motion. Static stability is provided by the joint capsule, the glenoid labrum and the capsula-labral ligaments, which for the most part, are thickenings of the undersurface or internal surface of the anterior and inferior capsule and act as restraints or buttresses to excessive motion when throwing. These restraints are tested both in the sitting and supine position.

The sulcus sign refers to a visible depression on the lateral aspect of the shoulder, just lateral to the acromion. It is measured as +, , +, which refers to the millimeters of gap 5–10, 10–15, greater than 15. Looser shoulders, in particular those with what is referred to as multi-directional instability, will show an obviously positive sulcus sign and a great deal of excursion — front-to-back, and vice versa when pressure is applied to the humeral head from each direction. This can be palpated with the athlete sitting and his elbow to forearm resting on the examiner's knee, or with the player lying supine with his or her shoulder at the edge of the examining table. When in the supine position, the test is more accurately carried out if the joint is preloaded at first — that is, the joint and pressure applied to the point of the elbow with the examiner's thigh while the shoulder is in 90 degrees of abduction and 90 degrees of external rotation.

5. **Diagnosis.**

Upper extremity

Shoulder Injuries — impingment of the rotator cuff beneath the coracoacromial arch can cause rotator cuff strain and/or tear, or tendinitis.

Other injuries can be tears of the glenoid labrum, many of which are due to associated instability.

History — Loss of velocity
    Loss of location of pitch
    "Deadarm"
    + clicking and popping

Examination — Look for sulcus sign

Sitting — stabilize scapular — more humeral head back and forth

    Jobe's relocation test — bring humeral head forward with shoulder abducted 90° and externally rotated maximum and if pain elicited in front of shoulder, push back on head of the humans and see if pain is relieved. Supine — load humeral head into glenoid and try to shift humeral head in each direction.

Imaging studies — M.R.I., in many instances, is too sensitive. Partial tears and tendinitis look the same. Two studies have shown 30% abnormality rate in asymptomatic shoulders.

 C.T. Arthrogram — arthrogram still good in looking at full thickness and undersurface partial thickness cuff tears. CT part of study is good for labral and capsular tears. If the joint takes large volume of air and contrast material, this signifies a loose capsule.

Arthroscopy — most direct way of evaluating cuff and labrum; wear on anterior labrum with or without complete tear.

Labral tears —
   History — frequently associated with instability symptoms.
   Examination — clunk test for posterior labrum.
   Patient supine — try to piston humeral head posteriorly and feel for "clunk".
   Sitting with hands on hips — try to apply axial pressure from elbow up through shoulder. Imaging studies — see above.
   Arthroscopy — can evaluate entire 360 degrees of labrum.
Biceps strain (tendinitis) —
   History — overuse strain. Tight when first warming up and becomes looser. Aching the following day. Responds quickly to rest.
   Examination — can reproduce pain by palpation in bicipital groove. Can provoke pain by supination of forearm against resistance or flexion of shoulder against resistance.

TREATMENT OF SHOULDER INJURIES

It is important to bear in mind that following any surgical procedures on the throwing shoulder — even simple trimming of a partial rotator cuff tear or labrum — that it can take 8–10 months before the athlete is able to "air it out" and throw 100%. Many of the exercise programs outlined in Chapter 2 done properly and with patience can lead to the same result without surgery.

Occasionally, a subacromial injection of a corticosterioid (Cortisone), along with rest, will be all that is needed.

TREATMENT OF ELBOW INJURIES

The following conditions can occur in the region of the elbows as a result of excessive throwing:

Management of Baseball Injuries

Strain of the joint capsule, ligaments or surrounding muscles
Swelling due to inflammation of the lining of the joint
Posterior compartment spurs- bone spurs along the edges of the bones on the back of the elbow
Ulnar nerve irritation alone, or associated with
Ulnar collateral ligament strains or tear — these lesions along with posterior compartment spurs result from the so called "valgus overload syndrome" that results from the excessive opening up of the inner side of the joint during the cocking action of throwing
Growth center abnormalities — partial complete separation of the medial epicondyl in the skeletally immature player
Loose bodies — cartilage or bone fragments that break off and float freely about the elbow joint

The symptoms that can result from the aforementioned pathology can present as pain, tightness, popping and clicking, swelling or locking of the joint. Any one or all of these symptoms may be present.

Most of these injuries occur in the act of throwing. There is tension applied to the medial (inner) side of the elbow and compression to the lateral (outer) side of the elbow (diagrams). Therefore, the ulnar collateral ligament and the ulnar nerve and flexor-pronator muscle-tendon which originates on the medial condyle of the elbow is repeatedly stretched to the point where microtrauma may eventually lead to a complete tear (the feeling of a POP). The repeated compression on outer side of the elbow can cause deterioration of the joint surfaces between the capitellum of the humerus and the radial head. Ulnar nerve symptoms consist of a burning type pain on the inner aspect of the forearm and numbness and tingling in the 4th and 5th fingers (pinky) of the hand. The same injury to the medial collateral ligament of the inside of the elbow will cause a separation of the growth plate in the skeletally immature thrower (the medial epicondyle).

Symptoms — pain
                Tightness
                Popping and clicking
                Locking

The physician will relate the symptoms to underlying anatomy and pathology.

Pain may indicate — **Anterior** (antecubital) — must rule out thoracic outlet syndrome or median nerve compression.

lateral unlike racquet sports, lateral elbow pain is uncommon and when present is usually due to articular cartilage damage to the radiocapitellar joint due to valgus overload (i.e. compression).

posterior — triceps strain or tendinitis, olecranon spurs, olecranon – olecranon fossa joint surface, damage, synovitis.

medial — most common area of involvement — can be difficult to localize since the ulnar nerve, the common attachment of the pronator and wrist flexor to the medial epicondyle and the ulnar (medial) collateral ligament (the main medial stabilizer of the elbow) are all within 1–2 cm. of each other.

Tightness may indicate muscle fatigue or strain due to swelling within the joint. When the ulnar collateral ligament is inflamed or strained, the player may complain of tightness.

Popping and clicking may indicate loose bodies, the rubbing of tendons over bony prominences, or tears of ligaments and/or tendons. If in the act of throwing the player feels a sudden pop on the inner side of the elbow, this can be due to one of the following:

1. Subluxation of the ulnar nerve — this nerve is located on the inner side of the elbow ("the crazy bone") and is held in place by a very thin ligament. From repetitive throwing this can stretch out allowing the nerve to slide back and forth over the bone on the inside of the elbow and cause a sensation of popping during the act of throwing. Occasionally this can also be associated with a stinging or numbness of the 4th and 5th fingers.

2. A tear of the ulnar collateral ligament — usually with an acute tear during the acceleration and follow through phase of pitching the player may experience a pop on the inner side of the elbow. This is more commonly associated with trying to throw a slider more than most other pitches, although it can be seen with throwing a fastball.

3. A tear of the common pronator-flexor origin — this large tendon mass is just in front of the other structures and the same mechanism can cause it to tear, although more often this occurs in late follow through with any pitch as they all end with pronation of the forearm and some wrist flexion.

Diagnosis. This is made by the history and physical examination. Plain x-rays will show bone spurs and epiphyseal (growth center) separation, especially when compared to the opposite elbow. CAT Scans will show cartilaginous loose bodies. MRI is the best way to show tears of the major ligaments and/or tendons.

Treatment. Obviously, rest is the first line of treatment. With tears and epiphyseal separation, sometimes a decision needs to be made as to whether or not surgery is required to stabilize the area. Many of these less severe injuries will respond to three weeks of rest and non-steroidal anti-inflammatory drugs. Physical therapy is another treatment option.

Once the initial three weeks of non-surgical treatment is over, it will then be necessary to do strengthening exercises and get on a throwing program for another three weeks prior to competitive activity.

TREATMENT OF HAND AND WRIST INJURIES

Hand and wrist injuries are most commonly seen as a result of being struck by a pitched ball or falling on an outstretched hand. A ball striking the end of the finger can disrupt the extensor mechanism and this can result in a drop finger or mallet finger. When this type of injury occurs, the player is unable to actively extend (straighten) the DIP tip joint of the finger.

TREATMENT IF 1ST MP OR THUMB INJURIES

A common injury in all sports is the so Gamekeeper's thumb. This term describes a sprain of the ulnar collateral ligament of the MP joint of the thumb where the thumb joins the hand. This injury is due to a subacute stretching of the ligament; during athletic activity, a fall or a collision of the thumb with somebody else can cause the thumb to be driven away from the hand, resulting in this type of injury. There is tenderness and swelling at the metacarpal phalangeal joint. If there is major instability it usually requires surgical repair. If it is minor it can be treated with appropriate splinting and strapping.

TREATMENT OF WRIST INJURIES

Aside from direct trauma such as falls or being struck by a pitched ball, wrist injuries are more commonly caused by sliding into bases using the affected limb as a landing stabilizer. They are also caused by an abrupt checking of a bat swing. With advanced imaging techniques, many injuries that used to be passed off as sprains are now being found to be due to tears of the triangular fibrocartilage complex (TFCC). Pain and a sensation of "weakness" of the wrist during activity is usually the presenting complaint.

Other injuries of the wrist include ligament tears and scaphoid lunate dislocations.

TREATMENT OF HEAD AND NECK INJURIES

Injuries to the head and neck may occur in any sport. If a player loses consciousness it is the authors' belief that the patient should be removed from play and not allowed to resume play until evaluated by a physician over a course of several days. If a player suffers from dizziness, nausea, or has difficulty with memory, it is imperative that the patient be transported immediately for medical evaluation. With regard to head injuries, it is important to remember that any injury caused by a force severe enough to cause unconsciousness has the capability of causing a neck injury at the same time. Thus,

Management of Baseball Injuries

when someone suffers a severe head injury it is prudent to immobilize the neck until that player can be evaluated properly. Any severe injury to the neck itself1 should be treated with appropriate immobilization. If there is any significant sensory loss, that is loss of feeling anywhere, that player must be immobilized on the field prior to any transportation. If there are not trained personnel available, the best course of action is not to move the player until such time that emergency medical personnel arrive. This is a severe injury and can be made worse by ill-considered early motion of the patient. The neck should be stabilized and the patient's airway maintained as best as possible until trained help is available.

EXERCISE INDUCED ASTHMA (EIA)

About one in ten persons have asthma. In most cases, asthma is exhibited within the first 115 minutes of exercise. It is also referred to as exercise-induced bronchospasm (EIB). The term bronchospasm refers to the constriction of the air passages in the tracheobronchial tree. EIB is also exacerbated during exercise in cold weather. The most relevant symptoms include breathlessness, coughing, and wheezing. At the onset of such symptoms, the athlete should be removed from playing, rested, and the player's anxiety lowered. At a later time, if the coach, the athlete, or parent is confronted with these symptoms after a short interval of exercise, the athlete should consult a physician to check for asthma. In no way should asthma prevent a player from enjoying baseball. There are several therapeutic measures the physician usually prescribes. Among them—a prolonged warm-up time in order to reduce bronchoconstriction. The physician may prescribe inhalers with a short or long term bronchodilation effect. Some inhalers can be used within 15 minutes before exercise and/or days before exercise.

FURTHER GENERAL READING

Knight K.L. (1985) Cryotherapy Theory, Technique and Physiology. Chattanooga Corporation, Chattanooga, Tennessee.

Kellett J. (1986). Acute Soft Tissue Injuries — A Review of the Literature. Med. Sci. in Sports Exerc. 18:489–500.

Landry G.L. and Gomez J.E. (1991). Management of Soft Tissue Injuries. In Adol. Med. State of the Art Revs. 2:125–140.

Bocobo C. et al. (1991). The Effect of Ice on Intra-articular Temperature in the Knee of the Dog. Am. J. of Phys. and Med. Rehab. 70:181–5

Belitsky R.B. et al. (1987). Evaluation of the Effectiveness of Wet Ice, Dry Ice, and Cryogenic Packs in Reducing Skin Temperature. Phys. Therapy, 67:1080–4.

Clarkson P.M. et al. (1992). Muscle Function After Exercise-Induced Muscle Damage and Rapid Adaptation. Med. and Sci. in Sports and Exerc. 24:512–520.

Mahler, Donald A. (1993). Exercise-induced asthma. Med. Sci. Sports Exerc., 25:554–561.

Chapter FOUR

Water and Electrolyte Balance for Baseball Players

Water is the most important nutrient for the baseball player before, during, and after the game. During exercise, all of the energy expenditure leads to a large amount of heat production. Evaporation of water through the skin (i.e., sweating) is the critical avenue for cooling and maintaining the core body temperature. The evaporated water which is lost should be replenished in order to restore the normal blood and cellular ionic concentrations which are vital to normal functions. In addition, drinking cold water can cool the body and maintain it at 37°C. The player should drink 1–2 glasses of cold water two hours prior to the practice/game. Also, the player should drink 1 glass of water for every 1 lb weight loss during a practice/game. During the practice/game, the player should drink 4–6 ounces of water every 15–20 minutes to insure proper hydration and well being. If the body temperature is not maintained at 37°C, the following heat-related illnesses (in order of increasing seriousness) can occur: heat cramps, heat exhaustion, and heat stroke.

Water is the most critical nutrient for the survival and well being of a person. One can survive without the intake of other nutrients for days, weeks, and even months but one cannot survive without water for more than a few days. In a 70 kg (154 lb) person, the water content is about 40 liters (10.56 gallons) (i.e., 60% of body weight). Most of the water (25 liters) is inside cells; nevertheless, about 15 liters reside outside of cells. The blood volume is about 5 liters (1.32 gallons) and the maintenance of this volume is critical to a person's survival, despite the fact that daily fluid intake can vary from 1–8 liters. Excess fluid intake can easily be regulated; however, a problem arises when fluid intake is below one liter per day and blood volume starts to decrease below 5 liters (for example, a blood volume of 4 liters or less can cause death). Under sedentary conditions the skin and the kidneys (i.e., urine output) are the most important regulators of body water. Under conditions of hot weather and exercise (despite fluid intake in many cases), the skin because of sweating) becomes the only important regulator of body water, as well as body temperature. Loss of water in a heavy, prolonged exercise (e.g., a 3 hour marathon) can increase from 0.1 to 5 liters.

Sweating is an absolute necessity in maintaining constant body temperature. The sweat rate usually corresponds to increases in energy expenditure by the athlete. Trained athletes have more sensitive sweating systems than non-athletes due to adaptation to repetitive exercise. For example, a marathon runner's fluid losses (despite fluid intake in many cases) can consist of 12% of body water and 8% of body weight. Greater than 1% weight loss secondary to water loss from exercise induces severe demands on the thermoregulatory and cardiovascular systems. Fluid losses during adult baseball games can range from less than 1% to 3% of body weight. Obviously, such a loss should be dealt with in a serious manner.

Water and Electrolyte Balance

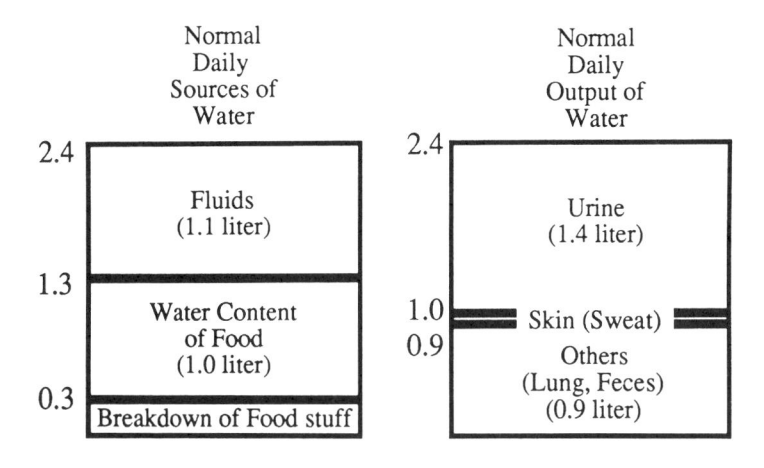

```
            Normal                    Normal
            Daily                     Daily
            Sources of                Output of
            Water                     Water
    2.4  ┌─────────────────┐   2.4  ┌─────────────────┐
         │     Fluids      │        │     Urine       │
         │   (1.1 liter)   │        │   (1.4 liter)   │
    1.3  ├─────────────────┤        │                 │
         │  Water Content  │   1.0  ├═════════════════┤
         │    of Food      │   0.9  │  Skin (Sweat)   │
         │   (1.0 liter)   │        │     Others      │
    0.3  ├─────────────────┤        │  (Lung, Feces)  │
         │Breakdown of Food stuff│  │   (0.9 liter)   │
         └─────────────────┘        └─────────────────┘
```

Figure 4.1. An example of the daily amount in liters of water intake (first bar) and output (second bar) for a sedentary person. The numbers given are approximate guesses for normal environmental conditions of temperature and humidity.

All of the energy expenditure during exercise results in heat. Therefore, body temperature will rise rapidly during exercise if cooling due to sweating does not occur. The prolonged increase in body temperature will eventually cause serious damage to the thermoregulatory system, which can result in serious damage to the body's most sensitive organ — the brain. Also, even moderate dehydration could contribute to changes in mental status and increased muscle injuries. Thirst, unfortunately, is not a reliable indicator of water loss or rise in body temperature during exercise (or under any stressful condition, particularly in young athletes). Therefore, athletes should drink water not just to quench their thirst, but as part of their exercise regime. Figures 4.1 and 4.2 represent a hypothetical daily water output and water intake for people who are sedentary, who have run a 3 hour marathon, or are playing baseball (90–100 minutes). The numbers are rough estimates, and are only for illustrative purposes. The most scientific way to determine optimal water intake is to weigh the player before and during the game. The loss of weight due to water loss should be adjusted by drinking the same amount

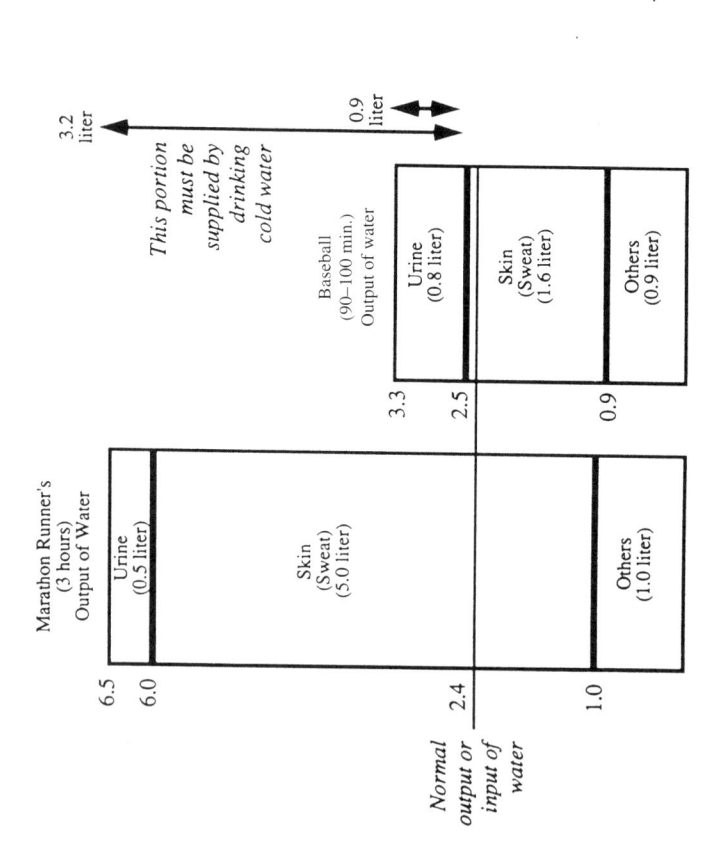

Figure 4.2. An example of the daily required amounts in liters of water needed to be consumed by a marathon runner (3 hours) and a baseball player (90–100 minutes). The values given are rough estimates for normal environmental conditions of temperature and humidity.

of water. Remember, it is better to drink more than less water. The athlete should drink 1–2 glasses of water two hours before the practice/game and 1 glass of water for every 1 lb weight loss during the event. Alternatively, the athlete could do well by simply drinking 4–6 ounces of water every 15–20 minutes during the event. The water should be cold for two reasons; cold water provides a greater capacity to lower core body temperature and it quickens the emptying of the stomach content into the intestines where water absorption occurs.

Children utilize more metabolic energy than adults in performing the same task, and thus they produce more heat. Fortunately, children dissipate heat more efficiently than adults due to a larger surface area to mass ratio. However, the surface area to mass ratio advantage for children is offset by the fact that children have less sweating capacity than adults. When the ambient temperature is hot and humid, the dissipation of heat is inhibited and thus children may be at a greater risk of heat related illnesses than adults during exercise.

Electrolytes such as Na^+, K^+, Cl^-, Ca^{2+}, and Mg^{2+} are very important ions and their concentrations in the cell and blood are critical for maintaining normal body function. As we sweat more during exercise, the amount of these ions in the sweat is less than that of the blood. In other words, the body is losing more water than ions. Under heavy exercise conditions, the body loses about 5–7 grams of sodium chloride. However, there is a minimal loss of K^+ and Mg^{2+}. Under conditions of continued exercise (up to 60 minutes) there is a need to replenish water continuously, but not salt. If there is heavy exercise beyond the 60 minutes, salt and carbohydrate replenishment is appropriate. 2–4 glasses of about 6% carbohydrate solution is recommended. The use of salt tablets during the early phase of exercise (as in most cases of baseball) is detrimental to the body. The body fluid has a higher salt concentration after exercise than before; therefore, the body needs pure water to bring the blood composition back to normal levels. The presence of ions in drinking water may slightly facilitate water absorption through the intestines and its retention in the body. It is because of this fact and the salt replacement in a prolong exercise that "sport drinks" advocates (primarily companies that sell them) promote drinking "sport drinks" for rehydration. However, since the health risks from dehydration far outweighs the risks taken because of a small amount of salt depletion (not present in most youth baseball players due to the limited amount of true activities), it is therefore of paramount importance to first ensure proper hydration with water. However, if the player has two games per day (such as in tournaments), it is then advisable to drink juices or "sports drinks" which contain salt, particularly after each game. After practice/game, the baseball player should ingest large amounts of carbohydrates in order to replenish muscle glycogen content. The ingestion of carbohydrates within the first two hours after play is preferred because it is at this time that muscles have an enhanced capacity to synthesize glycogen. Calcium supplementation maybe needed especially for female athletes if blood calcium levels are low.

HEAT RELATED ILLNESSES

Heat Cramps

Heat cramps are similar to other muscle cramps, and may be due to sudden blows, over exercise, lack of blood supply, etc.

Cause: Reduced blood flow to the muscle due to: loss of water, prolonged loss of minerals, etc.

Symptoms: Spasmodic tonic contraction of a given muscle (e.g., abdominal and extremities).

Onset: Gradual or sudden.

Danger: None if treated. Heat cramps could lead to termination of that particular exercise for a few days.

Prevention: Proper physical fitness, proper warm-ups and stretching exercises prior to the activity, and proper hydration.

Treatment: Termination of activity. Stretching, rest and ice treatment necessary.

Heat Exhaustion

Cause: Loss of water.

Symptoms: Tiredness, weakness, malaise, and feeling progressively weaker, anxiety, dizziness, at times fainting, and hot/dry skin. Persons will experience sweating, a small urine volume, and perhaps unconsciousness.

Onset: Gradual; over several days.

Danger: Rarely, the player may go into shock because of reduced blood volume. However, typically heat exhaustion is not an emergency condition. If not treated, this illness can lead to heat stroke.

Prevention: Proper physical fitness and proper hydration before and during exercise.

Treatment: Termination of activity, rest in a recumbent position cooling down, drinking water, and later drinking large amounts of mineral rich fluid such as diluted (1:3) fruit and vegetable juices.

Heat Stroke

Brain cells in the hypothalamus maintain body temperature close to 37°C (98.6°F). These cells respond to the blood temperature that passes through them. The cells regulate body temperature by sending signals to release skin vasodilators in order to increase sweating. When rectal temperatures reach 41°C–43°C, unconsciousness may occur; if that happens, the mortality rate ranges from 50–70%. Heat stroke is the second biggest cause of death after accidental death among athletes. In a recent August, 1996 story, 14 Mexican troops died in training exercise (The Washington Post., August 3, 1996, p. A 24).

Cause: Loss of water and a sudden uncontrolled rise in body temperature due to the failure of the thermoregulatory center in the brain.

Symptoms: Heat stroke should be treated as a life threatening *Medical Emergency* as it may lead to death or irreversible brain damage. The person shows behavioral or mental status changes during heat stress. These symptoms include: a sense of impending doom, headache, dizziness, confusion, hysteria, and weakness. The person exhibits hot and dry skin, rapid pulse, and low blood pressure. Factors which could lead to heat stroke include:

    a.   environmental high temperature and high humidity.
    b.   high rectal temperature.

c. hot dry skin (i.e., sweating stops).
   d. cardiorespiratory (e.g., rapid weak pulse, low blood pressure) and central nervous system disturbances.
   e. clouded consciousness and finally, collapse.

Onset: Sudden.

Danger: Brain damage and death is imminent if not treated quickly.

Prevention: Proper physical fitness and proper hydration before and during the exercise.

Treatment:

1. Call for an ambulance.
2. Remove clothes and cool with ice and cold water on the body.
3. Monitor vital signs (i.e., breathing, heart beat, pupil size).
4. Massage extremities to promote cooling.
5. Once the body temperature cools and the person is quite alert, remove from cold environment to prevent hypothermia.
6. Do not attempt to force water on an unconscious individual as they will choke on it.

In the hospital, the personnel may perform the following:

1. Administer I.V. fluid (perhaps 2–3 liters for 1st hour depending on blood pressure and pulse).
2. Monitor urinary output — Mannitol may be given to promote urination.
3. Digitalis may be given in cases where heart failure is a possibility.
4. Possible administration of medication to increase cardiac output (if needed).
5. Oxygen may be given.
6. Other procedures as necessary may be used.
7. Continue to monitor kidney and brain functions, and vital signs.

Figure 4.3 represents a flow diagram which summarizes how the various heat related illnesses can result from heat stress. It is important for the readers to realize that once the athlete undergoes a bout of heat exhaustion or heat stroke, he/she may have damaged their thermoregulatory system. The thermoregulatory system has a set point of 37°C, but the damaged thermoregulatory system may have a higher set point and thus the athlete may become susceptible to bouts of heat related illness and can further damage the thermoregulatory system. Therefore, it is important for the athlete to exercise preventive measures in order to reduce the chances of heat related illnesses.

Heat Illness Chart

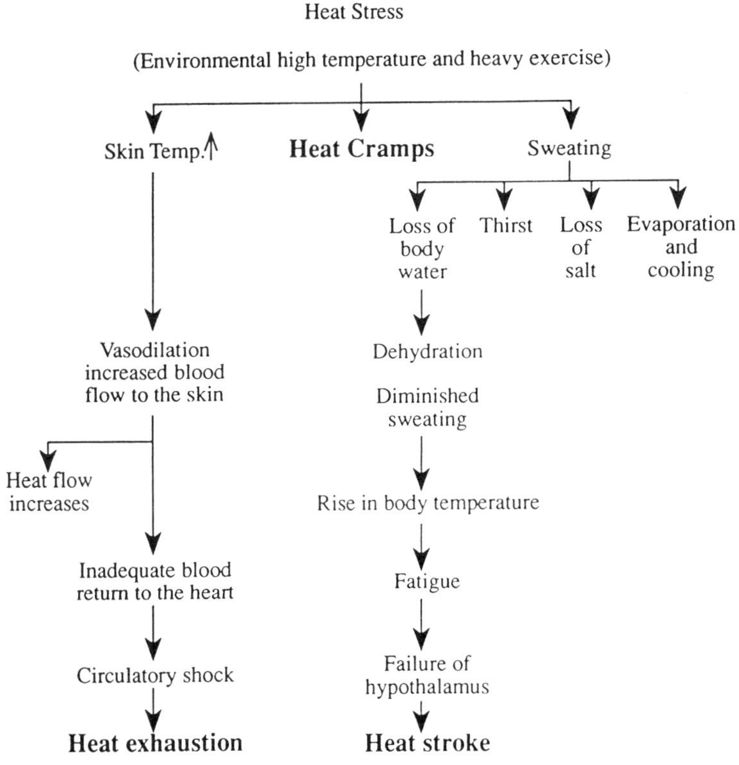

Heat Stress

(Environmental high temperature and heavy exercise)

```
              ↓              ↓                    ↓
         Skin Temp.↑   Heat Cramps            Sweating
              │              │                    │
              │      ┌───────┼───────┬────────────┐
              │      ↓       ↓       ↓            ↓
              │   Loss of  Thirst  Loss      Evaporation
              │    body            of            and
              │   water            salt        cooling
              │      │
              ↓      ↓
        Vasodilation   Dehydration
        increased blood
        flow to the skin
              │       │
              │       ↓
              │   Diminished
              │    sweating
     ┌────────┤       │
     ↓        │       ↓
  Heat flow   │   Rise in body temperature
  increases   │       │
              │       ↓
              ↓     Fatigue
        Inadequate blood  │
        return to the heart
              │       ↓
              ↓    Failure of
        Circulatory shock  hypothalamus
              │       │
              ↓       ↓
        Heat exhaustion   Heat stroke
```

Figure 4.3. Flowchart of heat related illnesses and the relevant pathways that lead to heat cramps, heat exhaustion, and heat stroke.

FURTHER GENERAL READING

Barr S.I. et al. (1990). Fluid Replacement During Prolonged Exercise: Effects of Water, Saline, or No Fluid. Med. Sci. Sports Exerc. 23:811–817.

Coyle E.F. et al. (1983). Carbohydrate Feeding During Prolonged Strenuous Exercise Can Delay Fatigue. J. of Appl. Phys. 55:230–235.

American College of Sport Medicine (1996), Position Stand, "Exercise and Fluid Replacement" Med. Sci. Sports Exerc., 28:i–vii.

Chapter FIVE

Adaptation to Endurance Training

Endurance training connotes a process of adaptive changes to achieve the strength, power, and cardiorespiratory capacity necessary in order to complete a specific physical task. Endurance training requires several months of rhythmic and continued exercise, and results in an increase in the body's number of capillaries, maximal oxygen uptake, stroke volume, and muscle enzymes. Moreover, endurance training increases the sectional size of slow type fibers. There can be also be an actual conversion of fast type fibers Type IIB (Type 2B) to fast Type IIA (Type 2A) to slow Type I. The Type IIB fibers are capable of lasting longer than the Type IIA fibers while Type I fibers are slow and long lasting like those of a marathon runner. Therefore, there are major underlying biochemical changes in the various organs and cells involved in the physical activity that provides the needed energy, strength, and power to carry out specific tasks. Baseball requires a combination of slow and fast fibers because playing baseball is a combination of quick actions lasting less than 1 minute and prolonged activities which can last 1–3 minutes.

Understanding endurance training has become a very serious scientific endeavor. In the past twenty years, there has been an increase in our understanding of the physiology and biochemistry of exercise. There has also been an increase in interest in the mechanism of how exercise induces physiological and biochemical adaptation at the cellular and organ level and how this accounts for the improved performance of athletes in a given sport. In an oversimplified way, we can view exercise as a transient damage to the tissue that stimulates repair beyond the original level. In this context, a prolonged resting period between bouts of exercise is essential for full repair of muscle tissue.

Endurance in sports means the ability of the person to perform a specific prolonged exercise or type of work, in order to achieve a reasonable goal without adverse reactions such as fatigue, exhaustion, or injury. Endurance can mean different things for different tasks (ex. Sport activity), as each task may involve unique muscle groups and skill levels. Therefore, there are several components of endurance that develop differentially during repetitive endurance training for a specific sport. The components which contribute to increased endurance are: **muscle strength and power, the cardiovasculatory system, and the respiratory system**. Cardiorespiratory endurance requires varying intensities in different sports. However, strength and power can vary in magnitude from muscle to muscle. Therefore, local or regional muscle group endurance is quite important for a given sport. During an endurance training period consisting of repetitive exercise for several months, the muscles adapt to generate force and to maintain a supply of energy. The key factor in endurance training is the exertion of physical stress with certain frequency and for variable lengths of time. This chronic muscular activity stimulates growth of the muscle as well as the development of endurance in terms of oxygen delivery, energy production, and permanent metabolic and structural changes. Therefore, endurance training in this context is a low level, prolonged intensity, aerobic training type of exercise where the system can utilize oxygen as the initial trigger of energy source. In general, the first aspect of endurance adaptation is the adaptation of the cardiovascular — respiratory system to accommodate the increased demand for oxygen uptake and delivery.

CARDIOVASCULAR-RESPIRATORY ADAPTATION

Rhythmic and continued exercise requires a greater use of oxygen at the muscle site. Therefore, the routes of uptake and transport of oxygen from the air to muscle tissues must adapt to take increased rate of delivery and extraction. A measurement of cardiorespiratory endurance is the VO_2max. VO_2max, which differs from person to person, is a measurement of the maximal oxygen uptake during the maximal exercise. In order to compare exercise-related data from person to person, the data are expressed relative to a specific level of intensity of exercise and expressed as a percent of VO_2max. To illustrate its importance, endurance training can change the VO_2max by as much as 20%. This is the first indication that true structural and biochemical changes must occur in order to metabolize the increased oxygen uptake. The first apparent result of exercise is the immediate increase in heart rate. The average resting heart rate is about 80 beats per min; however, during exercise the heart rate can go as high as 190 beats per min. After several months of endurance training heart rates in resting states can go as low as 40 beats per min. This reflects several factors of adaptation to exercise, one of them being the autonomic nervous system. However, despite the lowered heart rate, the heart still provides a greater cardiac output. This is because the volume of blood pumped per beat or stroke volume increases by as much as 80%. In a highly trained athlete, the refilling of the heart with return blood is more complete. More importantly, the left ventricle strength and power is dramatically increased. The left ventricle undergoes hypertrophy with endurance training, due to increased heart muscle mass and volume. Heart size is greater in an endurance trained athlete by as much as 25%, as compared to a sedentary person. Moreover, the amount of contractile proteins is increased and the composition of these contractile proteins are changed. Also, oxygen delivery of the blood supply to the heart is improved because the number and size of capillaries per cross-sectional area of muscle increases by as much as 50% due to endurance training. Endurance training also improves (by as much as 80%) the muscle content of myoglobin, a protein which carries oxygen within the muscle tissue. These dramatic biochemical adaptations in the oxygen delivery system parallel those of the heart and thus complements the entire scope of the biochemical adaptation which results in a better performance by the trained athlete.

BLOOD VOLUME AND COMPOSITION

There are three major changes in the blood due to endurance training: (1) increased blood volume; (2) increased hematocrit (i.e., increase in the total number of red blood cells (RBC)); and (3) decreased blood viscosity. The increased blood volume is as high as 20%. However, the increase in RBC mass is less pronounced and as a consequence the viscosity of the blood decreases. The increase in blood volume is of primary importance for the endurance trained athlete. The increased blood volume enhances O_2 delivery as well as enhancing microcirculation (i.e., small capillaries within muscle). The increase in microcirculation is even more pronounced due to the blood's reduced viscosity. The trained athlete also has another advantage in the greater capacity to clear lactate from the muscle and utilize lactate as an energy substrate. Thus, the level of blood lactate in a trained athlete is lower than that of the sedentary person. This phenomenon is referred to as the lactate shift. A trained athlete, therefore, has greater endurance with less fatigue and cramps due to decreased levels of blood lactate.

ENERGY SOURCE

The direct energy source in cells is adenosine triphosphate (ATP). ATP is produced by the mitochondrial (the mitochondria is the powerhouse of the cell) enzymes. The Krebs cycle utilizes oxygen (an aerobic process) (also referred to it as oxidation) in the production of ATP. In order to utilize larger amounts of oxygen to produce more and more ATP for the trained athlete, the number of mitochondria increases by over 100% and the size of each mitochondria increases by as much as 35%. Therefore, there is a concomitant increase in all of the enzymes involved. A trained athlete develops the ability to store in skeletal muscle a greater amount of glycogen (up to 40% more) and triglycerides (a type of fat) (1.8%) than an untrained one. Another advantage for a trained athlete is the increased ability to utilize free fatty acids by as much as 30%. This increase in free fatty acids use results in sparing glycogen for later use if needed. The increased use of free fatty acids is consistent with the increased fatty acid oxidation enzymes in the endurance trained athlete.

MUSCLE FIBER COMPOSITION

The motor unit is considered the terminal functional element responsible for movement. Even though the distinctions among the three types of units is somewhat arbitrary, they serve as an initial handle in understanding the complex number of muscles involved in endurance training induced adaptation. Initial amounts of types of fibers are genetically predetermined. The "type 1" fibers are also called "slow — relaxing" or slow twitch. The "type 2" fibers are also called "fast — relaxing" or fast twitch. Type 2 fibers are classified into two major classes — type 2A and type 2B. Type 2B fibers "tend" (not in all cases) to represent the fast glycolytic (FG) (indicating quick utilization of glucose and stored glycogen during anaerobic process) and type 2A "tend" (not in all cases) to represent the fast oxidative-glycolytic (FOG) (indicating the utilization of oxidative process of Krebs cycle during aerobic process). There are also type 2C fibers that are considered intermediate between type 1 and type 2. Endurance exercise

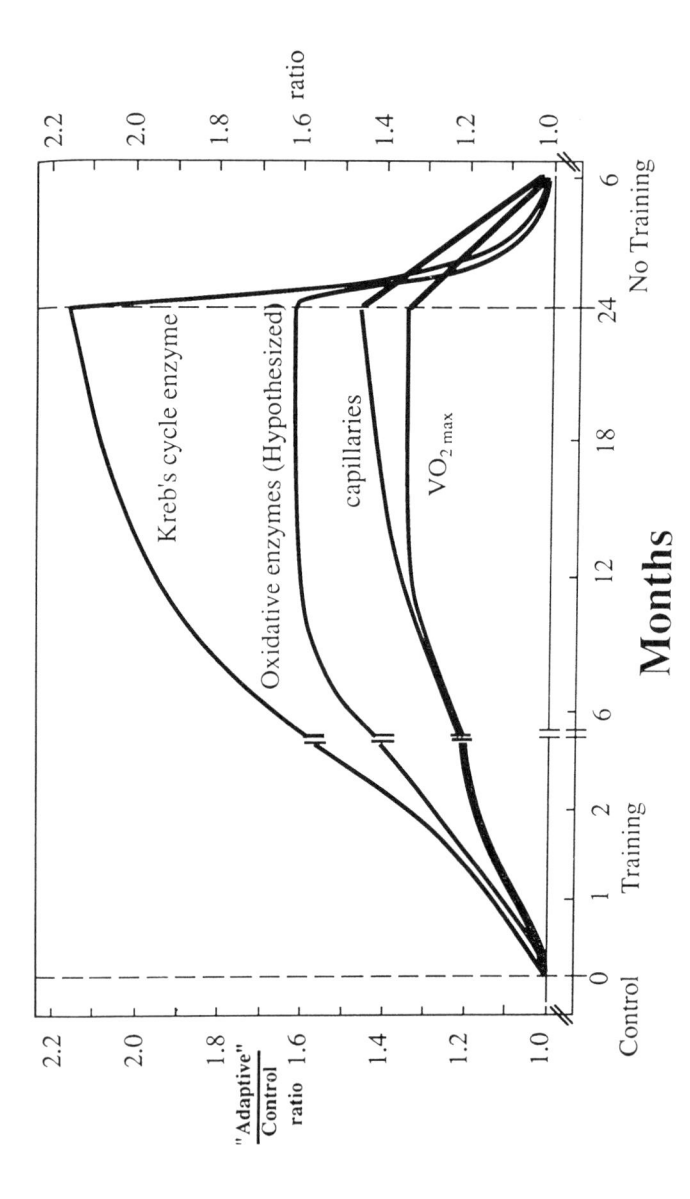

Figure 5.1. A schematic representation of the ratio of adaptation to control in man due to exercise based on data and hypothetical considerations for illustrative purposes. The figure is reproduced with permission from the publisher and the authors, Saltin et al., *Ann. N.Y. Acad. Sci.* 301:3–29, 1977. The curve on oxidative enzymes (hypothesized) was made by the authors.

causes changes from type 2B to type 2A to type 1 (i.e., towards slower and more long lasting fibers) with concomitant changes in the amount of enzymes. However, there are little and controversial evidence that slow twitch type 1 fibers can convert to fast twitch type II fibers. Endurance training also causes changes in the calcium regulatory enzymes in order to accommodate the new type of fibers. It is estimated that about a third of population's type 1 fibers can be influenced by exercise.

The adaptive process due to endurance training continues for up to six months beyond which little change occurs (see Figures 5.1 and 5.2). The cardiorespiratory parameters (VO_2, number of capillaries, enzymes), all increase in parallel in response to endurance training. However, increases in the muscle fiber conversion and the cross-sectional size occurs in a shorter time period (i.e., 1–2 months). Unfortunately, an absence of training results in a rapid decline of increased parameters to near control levels in 1–3 months. One exception may be the decline in the VO_2 and number of capillaries; in these cases, the decline is slower and may take about six months.

Baseball is a mixture of anaerobic and aerobic activities that requires endurance training and the use of slow fibers, and quick bursts of activity that requires anaerobic training and the use of fast fibers. In order to adapt the baseball player's muscles for the game, the athlete must consistently train both aerobically and anerobically for prolonged periods of time.

It is fortunate that once adaptation is achieved, the maintenance program is much less rigorous than the adaptation program. It appears that to induce adaptation in muscle cells, the intensity, frequency, and duration of training should be high compared to maintenance. Once endurance is achieved, the maintenance program can be as low as 40% of the intensity, frequency, and duration without a loss in endurance. This is important for young athletes since most of them do not participate in organized sports during the summer. Therefore, to maintain their achieved level of fitness and endurance, the athlete must perform a minimum of 2–3 workouts per week, consisting of 30–40 minutes of actually playing baseball or jogging and sprinting.

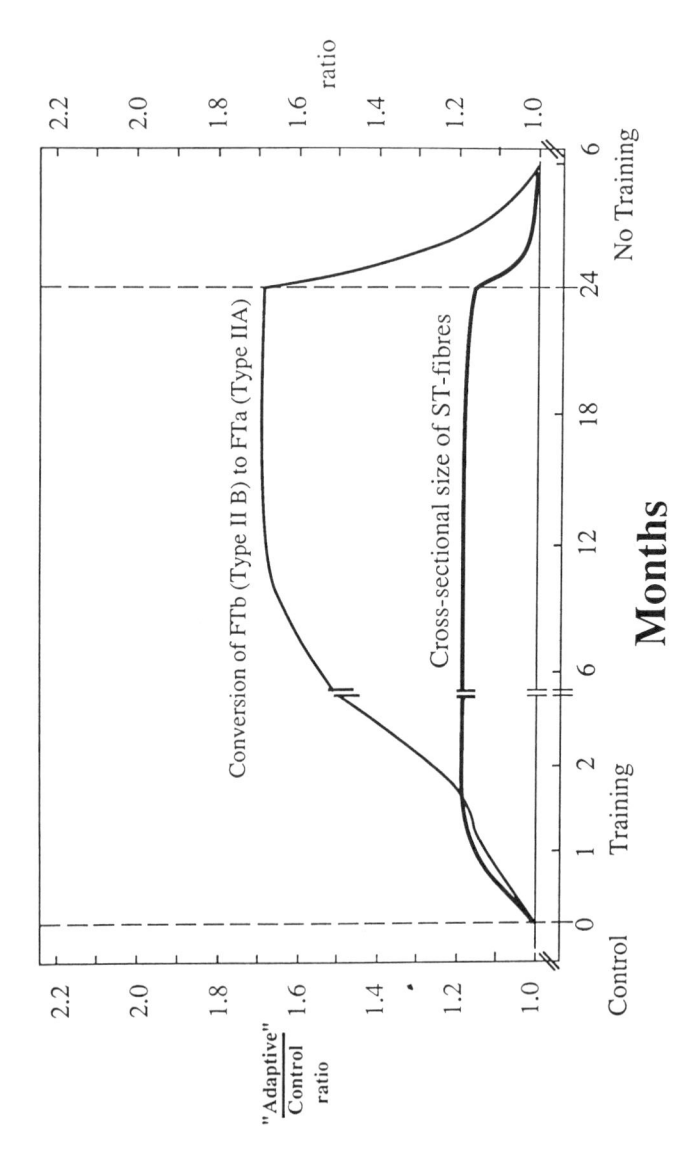

Figure 5.2. A schematic representation of the ratio of adaptation to control in man due to exercise based on data and hypothetical considerations for illustrative purposes. The figure is reproduced with permission form the publisher and the authors, Saltin et al., *Ann. N.Y. Acad. Sci.* 301:3–29, 1977.

FURTHER GENERAL READING

Anderson K.L. (1968). The Cardiovascular System in Exercise. In Exerc. Phys. H.B. Falls, editor, Academic Press, New York, USA.

Kjellberg S. et al. (1949). Increase of the Amount of Hemoglobin and Blood Volume in Connection with Physical Training. Acta Physiol. Cand. 19:146.

Klug G.A. and Tibbits G. F. (1988). The Effect of Activity on Calcium Mediated Entry in Striated Muscle. Exerc. Sports Sci. Rev. 16:1–159.

McArdle W.D. et al. (1991). Exercise Physiology. 3rd Edition, pp. 1–853. Lea & Febiger, Philadelphia (USA).

Saltin B. et al. (1977). Fiber Types and Metabolic Potentials of Skeletal Muscles in Sedentary Man and Endurance Runners. Ann. N.Y. Acad. Sci., 301:3–29.

Wilmore J.H. and Costill D.L. (1988). Training For Sport and Activity, 3rd edition, pp. 1–420, Wm. C. Brown Publishers, Dubuque, Iowa (USA).

Chapter SIX

Nutritional Requirement for Baseball Players

The most beneficial diet for a young baseball player involves eating balanced meals consisting of an average ratio of 5:1:1. of carbohydrates; proteins; fats. When exercising, the body primarily requires additional calories, and the best calories for an athlete to consume are in the form of carbohydrates. Increased exercise requires a proportional increase in the intake of carbohydrates. The pre-game meals should be primarily composed of carbohydrates, and balanced meals should be eaten prior to game days. Just prior to and during the game, the player should drink adequate amounts of cold water (2–3 glasses). In an ideal situation, the athlete during the event should drink 4–6 ounces of water every 15–20 minutes.

The human body is an organism which is composed of cells. Nutritional requirements are needed to maintain the normal cell functions in order to carry out the tasks which the body performs.

Like the rest of us, athletes, trainers, and coaches have a very limited knowledge of nutrition. Unfortunately, the societal pressures for winning induces athletes and others to invent the most bizarre concoctions of food which are then deemed proper "nutrition." These wild recipes are based on the most unscientific and the least documented studies. Most of these recipes are based on personal experiences associated with the food last eaten before a successful performance. For an athlete, a balanced diet should consist of three main constituents; carbohydrates, proteins, and fats, with a weight ratio of 5:1:1 (and a caloric ratio of about 3:1:1). Unfortunately, the current average American diet is composed of a weight ratio of 3:1:1 (with a caloric ratio of about 2:1:1). In other words, there is too much intake of fats and proteins and not enough intake of carbohydrates. Healthy and balanced nutritional intake by the individual will not only help the athlete but also will diminish the chances of developing coronary heart disease and becoming obese.

CARBOHYDRATES

Carbohydrates are composed of carbon, hydrogen, and oxygen. The simplest form of carbohydrate is the sugar glucose. Other examples of simple carbohydrates are fructose and galactose. Examples of some complex carbohydrates are starch (e.g., from potatoes) and cellulose (a source of dietary fiber). The average American currently consumes 50% of carbohydrates as simple sugars, mainly in the form of sucrose. However, sucrose causes a fluctuation in insulin secretion. Too much insulin in the blood may lead to low blood sugar (hypoglycemia). Low blood sugar could contribute to symptoms such as weakness, dizziness, and hunger sensations. None of these symptoms are beneficial to the athletes during their activities. Fructose (fruit sugar) is absorbed well in the intestine and does not stimulate insulin secretion. Thus it does not promote large fluctuations of blood sugar levels. As we have mentioned earlier, exercise suppresses insulin secretion. Therefore, sugar intake during exercise will not lead to low blood sugar.

Carbohydrates serve as the main source of energy for the body, and they also serve as an important source of metabolic by-products. These by-products are critical for many cell functions including protein sparing, fat utilization, and energy production.

1. **Protein Sparing**. Proteins, as we will see later, are the main building blocks needed for muscle maintenance, repair, and growth. Proteins can also serve as a source of energy when carbohydrates are low. When needed, glucose is actually formed from proteins as is the case in marathon running or any other prolonged exercise (greater than 90 minutes). Under these conditions, muscle proteins are degraded in order to provide a source of glucose. This actually causes a reduction in muscle content and in the process increases the concentration of nitrogen (from the degradation of proteins) excreted in the urine. Therefore, the maintenance of an adequate supply of carbohydrates or body stores of carbohydrates in the form of glycogen is important in reducing muscle breakdown.

2. **Carbohydrates as a Primer for Fat Utilization**. Carbohydrates in the body undergo metabolism (i.e., breakdown to smaller units) in order to release useful energy. Some of the breakdown products of carbohydrates are needed to break down fats and release their energy. Therefore, when insufficient carbohydrates exist, fatty acid breakdown becomes incomplete, which results in acidic body fluids; this is not conducive for normal function.

3. **Carbohydrates as a Source of Fuel for the Brain**. The brain (i.e., central nervous system) almost solely utilizes glucose as its source of energy. Under low carbohydrates conditions, the brain utilizes larger amounts of fats as a source of energy. Nevertheless, low blood glucose due to even modestly low carbohydrate levels could cause the symptoms of hypoglycemia mentioned earlier, and under extreme conditions could even cause irreversible brain damage. However, the brain can adapt by using fats as a source of energy within a week of experiencing low blood sugar.

4. **Exercise and Stored Energy**. Glucose and carbohydrates are the most likely sources of energy when there is an immediate demand, such as in anaerobic exercise (e.g. sprinting). However, endurance sports are aerobic in nature and they utilize the most efficient forms of metabolism (using oxygen) to break down sugar and carbohydrates which are then used as energy sources.

A carbohydrate-rich diet results in increased stores of muscle and liver glycogen. About 75% of glycogen is usually stored in muscle, about 20% in liver, and the remainder is stored in the blood. Glycogen stores are the critical factor that determines how long an athlete can exercise before becoming exhausted. There is a near linear relationship between the length of time an athlete can sustain an exercise, and the amount of stored glycogen which is used. Baseball players may become less (rarely) energetic during the last innings of play due to glycogen depletion in muscles. The ingestion of glucose polymers (series of glucose molecules hooked together) during exercise can prolong the exercise time to exhaustion. Moreover, glucose-polymers do not decrease the transit time of food in the intestine. The decrease in transit time in intestine would decrease absorption of the glucose-polymer. After an event, baseball players, just as other athletes, have low levels of muscle glycogen. Therefore, it is advisable for the athlete to ingest large quantities of carbohydrates within the first two hours after a game or practice. The muscle content of glycogen is very low following an event and thus there is an enhanced ability in the muscle to store glycogen. Baseball players should have high levels of muscle glycogen content before the game. Since the glycogen storage enzymes work much more efficiently after exercise, it is important that the athlete takes advantages of this enhanced proficiency by ingesting a large amount of carbohydrates after a game. In this way, the player will build up an adequate store of carbohydrates which can then be utilized at subsequent games. Obviously, adequate rest and proper food intake must accompany exercise.

PROTEINS

Proteins consist of carbon, oxygen, hydrogen, and nitrogen. Nitrogen is the distinct atom that is associated with proteins as compared to fats and carbohydrates which only consist of carbon, oxygen, and hydrogen. Also, proteins may contain sulfur, phosphorus, and iron. Proteins, which are large molecules made up of smaller molecules called amino acids, are required for numerous bodily functions. Among the most important body functions that involves proteins are enzymatic processes; transport; storage; the delivery of small molecules such as iron (Fe^{2+}, sodium (Na^+), potassium (K^+), calcium (Ca^{2+}) etc; muscle function (e.g., in skeletal and heart muscle); mechanical support (e.g., collagen in fibers); the immune system all antibodies against foreign invaders are proteins); nerve function (e.g., many neurotransmitters are proteins); and growth and differentiation (e.g., hormones, regulation of genes, etc). There are nine amino acids (called essential amino acids) which are not synthesized in the adult body, and must be provided through the intake of foods. The other eleven amino acids are synthesized in the body and thus need not be provided by a food source. These are called *non-essential amino acids*. The most important sources of proteins are meat, fish, poultry, eggs, and dairy products.

At the beginning of each heavy training season, serious athletes should increase their intake of proteins by almost 20–30%. This increased protein intake will compensate for the immediate need to increase muscle mass, and other amino acid-requiring proteins such as red blood cells and myoglobin (the oxygen carries in muscle). As we have mentioned earlier, it has been observed that prolonged exercise causes protein breakdown when carbohydrate reserves are low. Therefore, an athlete should have an abundance of glycogen stores in the muscle in order to prevent muscle wastage and to maintain peak performance levels. Glycogen stores are replenished by the intake of a sufficient amount of carbohydrates.

FATS

Fats, like carbohydrates, also consist of carbon, oxygen, and hydrogen. Also, fats may contain phosphorous, nitrogen, and other elements. Fats are required for numerous bodily functions; among the most important are: (1) energy stores (i.e., fats produce the energy currency of the body, ATP); (2) structure (e.g., all cell membranes are made of fats); (3) hormones (some are derived from fats); (4) intracellular messengers; (5) insulation (e.g., fats prevent body heat loss); and (6) vitamin delivery (fat-soluble vitamins such as A, D, E, and K are carried by fats through the bloodstream). Triglycerides are the large portion of fats in fat tissues and in muscle tissues.

Almost all fats which are required for bodily functions can be synthesized in the body, with linoleic acid being the only possible exception. Therefore, the concept of essential versus non-essential fats is not as well defined as for amino acids. However as mentioned earlier, fat intake is needed for the absorption of fat-soluble vitamins. Fats are derived from meat, fish, poultry, and dairy products (e.g., butter).

Fats represent by far the largest source of stored energy in the body. In moderate exercise, energy is equally derived from carbohydrates and fats. During longer exercises (> 1 hr), carbohydrate resources are depleted, and fat utilization increases to up to 80% of all energy required. Endurance athletes can utilize more fats at an earlier stage of exercise, and thus can save carbohydrates for later use. The use of caffeine also increases early use of fats as a source of energy.

In intense exercise, energy is derived solely from carbohydrates. Carbohydrates are the only source of fuel that can be quickly mobilized for intense bouts of activities.

Figure 6.1 summarizes the use of foodstuffs as a source of energy under aerobic and anaerobic conditions. Furthermore, the figure shows that exercise causes adaptation in the utilization of different amounts of the three sources of nutrition. Drugs and hormones similarly influence the ratio of utilization of these three sources of energy.

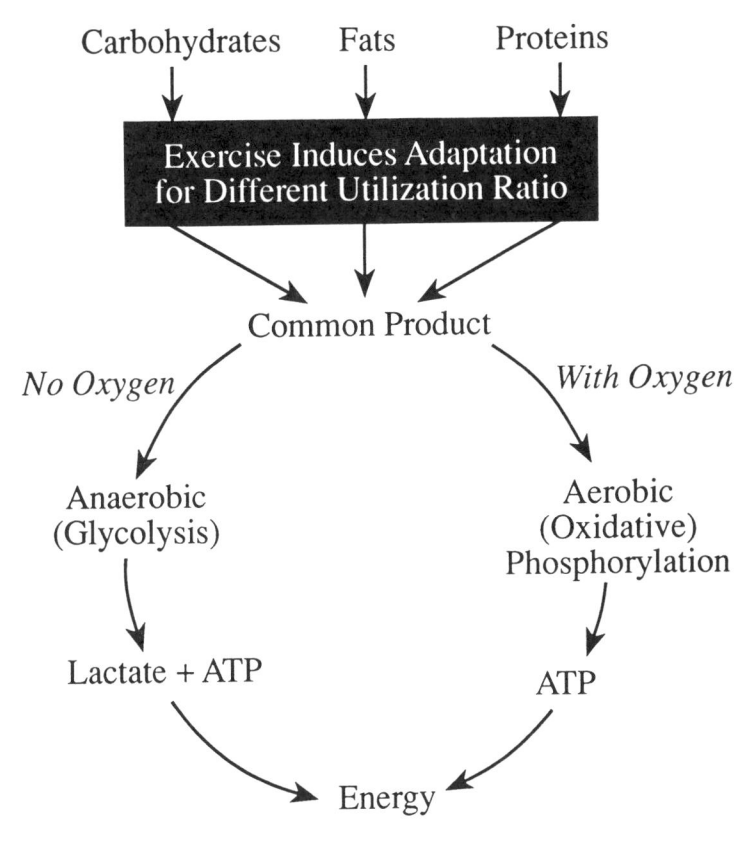

```
                Carbohydrates    Fats    Proteins
                      │           │         │
                      ▼           ▼         ▼
                ┌──────────────────────────────────┐
                │   Exercise Induces Adaptation    │
                │  for Different Utilization Ratio │
                └──────────────────────────────────┘
                                  │
                                  ▼
                          Common Product
                    No Oxygen /         \ With Oxygen
                            ▼             ▼
                       Anaerobic        Aerobic
                      (Glycolysis)     (Oxidative)
                                      Phosphorylation
                            │             │
                            ▼             ▼
                      Lactate + ATP      ATP
                             \           /
                              ▼         ▼
                               Energy
```

Figure 6.1. Flowchart of the metabolic pathways for foodstuff to energy production.

WATER AND ELECTROLYTES (see Chapter 5)

FOOD SUPPLEMENTS

Modern day literature has found that certain found supplements for athletes may contribute to optimal performance, especially for elite athletes. However, genetic predisposition, training, and mental preparation for the event play the largest role in optimal performance outcome. Moderate intake of carbohydrates as we maintained earlier is beneficial during the event. Also, moderate amounts of vitamins (one a day multivitamins for insurance) and antioxidants such as vitamin E, C (part of the multivitamins), beta-carotene, and selenium would be useful. There is a great deal of quakery and hype regarding sports food supplements. Over nutrition mega amounts could pose health risks to the athlete. Moderation is the message.

FURTHER GENERAL READING

Jones M. and Pedoe T. (1989). Blood Doping — A Literature Review. Brit. J. of Sports Med. 23:84–88.

Medical Commission of the International Olympic Committee (1989). Brit. J. of Sports Med. 23:60.

O'Neil F. et al. (1986). Research and Applications of Current Topics in Sports Nutrition. J. of the Am. Dietetic Ass. 86:1007–1015.

Inge K. and Garden L. (1990). Nutrition Advice for Athletes. Aust. Fam. Phy. 19:133–138.

Wolineky, I. And Hickson, Jr., J.F., Editors, (1994). "Nutrition in Exercise and Sport," 2nd edition, CRC Press, Boca Raton, Florida, pp. 1–416.

Chapter SEVEN

Drugs and Hormones in Sport

Unfortunately, there is a widespread use of drugs and hormones among athletes in order to try to enhance the accomplishment of short range goals. Examples of such drugs and hormones used are: steroids; growth hormones; amphetamines; and, the most seemingly benign of all of them, caffeine. Anabolic steroids in males (androgens or "male hormones") can cause stunted growth, testicular atrophy, liver damage, and increased breast size. In females, use of these same steroids can lead to male pattern baldness, deepening of the voice, unwanted hair patterns, enlargement of the clitoris, and dysfunction of the reproductive system and menstrual cycle. Growth hormone use can cause gigantism if given before the end of puberty, and can contribute to skin abnormalities, and enlarged bones. Amphetamine use can lead to addiction, headache, dizziness, confusion, anxiety, aggressiveness, impaired judgment, and may ultimately cause death. Caffeine use can spare carbohydrate depletion by the increased use of fats. However, because caffeine is a central nervous system stimulant, its heavy use can cause headaches, anxiety, insomnia, and increased urine output which can contribute to dehydration.

Athletes have always searched for a competitive edge over others using numerous ergogenic aids. Ergogenic aids connotes any agent (e.g., physical or nutritional etc....) that enhances performance. Great athletes have combined natural abilities, rigorous training, good coaching, and an outstanding competitive nature which enable them to achieve their competitive edge. Unfortunately, in modern times athletes have sought the use of biomedical knowledge about drugs and hormones in order to seek an unfair advantage. Aside from the unethical and illegal nature of the use of these drugs and hormones in sports, it is often dangerous to the athlete's own health and competitive edge. Moreover, these drugs, in addition to being dangerous, are illegal to use. Also, there is little documented scientific evidence that some of these drugs enhance performance. Therefore, the individual can significantly risk his/her health for an unsubstantiated and most likely detrimental effect of these drugs.

The following drugs and hormones will be discussed: steroids; growth hormones; amphetamines; and caffeine.

STEROIDS

The various types of steroids are either naturally occurring physiological steroid hormones or their synthetic analogues. All steroid hormones are derived from cholesterol. The relevant steroids about which the athlete should be aware of are called androgens. They produce an androgenic as well as an anabolic effect on the body. Androgenic effects are those effects which are related to male sexual maturation, and anabolic effects are those effects related to growth, such as an increase in mass and the rate of bone and muscle maturation.

The aim of synthetic steroids is to have compounds that selectively enhance anabolic effects without any androgenic effects. This is especially critical for female users. Heavy and prolonged steroid users can suffer from stunted growth due to early closure of the growth plates, liver damage, testicular atrophy, increased breast size (in males), and an increased risk of cardiovascular diseases.

Athletes use steroids to increase muscle mass and strength. Although there may be some evidence that steroids users have a greater muscle mass, the mechanism of increased muscle mass due to steroids use is not yet clear. Unfortunately, steroid users may gain some advantage in certain sports competitions; however, the risks far outweigh the benefits. Direct effects of steroids on muscle are controversial. It is thought that steroids use enhances the desire for more training and the ability to sustain more pain, in addition to a direct increase in muscle mass. Therefore, it is thought that steroids act on brain in a way which results in the desire for more frequent training that contributes to the eventual increase in muscle mass.

GROWTH HORMONE (GH)

GH is a naturally occurring hormone which is secreted by the pituitary gland. GH is involved in tissue growth by enhancing protein synthesis. Subsequently, this leads to an increased muscle mass and increased utilization of fats (for fuel), which spares carbohydrates. The fact that GH occurs naturally in the body is very attractive to athletes because they incorrectly assume that it is safe. However, prolonged and heavy use of GH in unphysiological quantities increases the risk of gigantism, skin abnormalities, oversized soft tissues, and enlarged bones. A further danger associated with the prolonged use of exogenous GH is the depression of physiological GH secretion. This decrease in normal physiological GH secretion can cause deleterious effects.

In addition, certain amino acids can temporarily enhance GH release. However, there is no strong evidence that the long term use of GH decreases body fat and increases muscle mass.

AMPHETAMINES

Amphetamines are prescription drugs which act as stimulants (also called "uppers") of the central nervous system (i.e., brain). Amphetamines reduce the sense of fatigue due to heavy exercise. The decrease in the sense of fatigue due to amphetamines is dangerous in itself because it inhibits our bodies' sense of when to slow down or stop a given exercise. Amphetamines also increase the following: vasoconstriction, blood sugar, pulse rate, breathing rate, and muscle tension. Amphetamines, therefore, act like the "fight and flight" hormones, ephinephrine and norephinephrine. The perception of enhanced performance in a specific sport, however, is not supported by the research data. The undocumented enhancement of performance due to amphetamines could lead to the deleterious side effects of the drug. The dangers associated with the use of amphetamines include; addiction, headaches, dizziness, confusion, increased reaction time, impaired judgement, anxiety, aggressiveness, insomnia, and possibly death with heavy usage.

CAFFEINE

Caffeine (methylxanthine) is a mild stimulant to the central nervous system. Caffeine is a natural component of coffee, tea, chocolate, etc. and acts as a stimulant to reduce the sense of fatigue due to exercise. Caffeine also increases the use of fats as fuel and thus spares carbohydrates which leads to added endurance for the athlete. Also, caffeine can increase the VO_2max; in addition, there is a small direct effect on the increased force of muscle contraction. Furthermore, caffeine can increase the availability of cellular calcium to the muscle. However, there are conflicting reports on the effect of caffeine on various physiological factors. Because caffeine is a stimulant, its use is associated with the following side effects; headaches, increased anxiety, insomnia, and increased urine output (diuresis) which can contribute to the dehydration of the athlete especially if combined with heavy exercise and in a hot environment.

FURTHER GENERAL READING

McNaughton L. (1987). Two Levels of Caffeine Ingestion on Blood Lactate and Free Fatty Acid Responses During Incremental Exercise. Res. Quar. for Exer. and Sport. 58(3):255–259.

Weir J. et al. (1987). A High Carbohydrate Diet Negates the Metabolic Effects of Caffeine During Exercise. Med. Sci. Sports Exer. 19: 100–105.

Sutton J. and Lazarus L. (1976). Growth Hormone in Exercise: Comparison of Physiological and Pharmacological Stimuli. J. Appl. Physiol. 41:523–527.

Crist D.M. et al. (1983). Effects of Androgen-Anabolic Steroids on Neuromuscular Power and Body Composition. J. Appl. Physiol. Respir. Environ. Exer. Physiol. 54(2):366–370.

Haupt H.A. and Rovere G.D. (1984). Anabolic Steroids: A Review of the Literature. Am. J. Sports Med. 12:469–484.

Lenders J.W. (1988). Deleterious Effects of Analogic Steroids on Serum Lipoproteins, Blood Pressure, and Liver Function in Amateur Body Builders. Int.. J. of Sports Med. 9(1):19–23.

Wilson J.D. and Griffin J.E. (1980). The Use and Misuse of Androgens. Metab. 29:1278–1295.

American Academy of Orthopedic Surgeons (1991). Athletic Training and Sports Medicine. Second Edition, American Academy of Orthopedic Surgeons, Park Ridge, Illinois.

Chapter EIGHT

Gender Difference and Skill Developlement

Recent evidence indicates that elite female athletes are catching up with elite male athletes. This new evidence supports the conviction among some people that the differences in athletic performances between the two genders are primarily due to outdated societal expectations and values. However, despite this new evidence, there are important physiological and biochemical differences that could contribute to different growths in skills and performance between males and females for a given sport. For example, the onset of puberty is about 2 years earlier in girls than in boys. Because of this, girls heights and weight is different from that of boys. Males usually have larger mass and greater aerobic power than females. However, puberty can also contribute to the delay in the acquisition of skills since are dependent on a sense of coordination coupled with the height and weight of the individual. Finally, female athletes may experience athletic amenorrhea (i.e. absence of their menstrual period). Athletic amenorrhea is associated with; low body fat, heavy exercise, poor nutrition, and genetic differences that influence the athlete's susceptibility to menstrual dysfunction.

There are obviously numerous physiological and biochemical differences between males and females. The real question is: are those physiological and biochemical differences the basis for some of the differences in performance in sports among males and females?

This is a highly controversial area. There are no clear cut answers at this time. The complicating factor has been that the societal expectations for performance in sports have been skewed in the past, (including the recent past) towards males. It is this important social factor that cannot be discounted when males out-perform females in certain sports. The recent federal Title IX which required that colleges offer similar sport programs to females as those offered to males, has resulted in large improvement of female athletic performance in all sports. The most recent research data indicates that the differences between genders is shrinking and this argues against inherent differences in abilities. Further support for this argument comes from the fact that present day elite female athletes in certain athletic events perform equal to or better than elite male athletes of just ten years ago.

Empirical observations indicate that boys usually perform better than girls in areas that require power and speed such as: running, jumping, and throwing. However, girls usually perform better than boys in areas that require balance such as hopping (i.e., dance and the like). These differences are augmented by the observation that on the average, VO_2max in boys is greater than girls and that boys have more anaerobic capability than girls.

Despite the above disclaimers in gender differences in athletic performance, there are important physiological, biochemical, and performance differences that have to be taken into consideration and dealt with in order to improve coaching and performance outcome in sports for both genders. We should note, however, that these differences between genders are insignificant before adolescence (puberty).

HEIGHT AND WEIGHT

In the first two years of adolescence, there is a high rate of growth in height and weight for both genders. Usually a girl's growth stops around 16 1/2 years old, and boy's growth stops around 18 years old. As we have mentioned in the summary, the onset of puberty is about 2 years earlier in girls than boys. Therefore, girls obtain full maturity of their bones earlier than boys. Bone growth is faster and more fully developed when it is subjected to exercise (i.e., moderate physical stress), as exercise is important for the tensile strength and diameter of the bone. The primary sites that determine height are at the growth plates (epiphyses) of the femur (upper leg). Therefore, proper treatment of injuries to growth plates is important in preventing the premature closure of these plates which can result in shorter stature.

MUSCLE

In both males and females, the mechanism of muscle adaptation due to exercise in terms of energy producing enzymes, fiber composition, and oxygen delivery, is the same. Full strength is fully attained at the age of 20 for females and between the ages of 20–30 in males. However, in males there is an increase in muscle mass due to testosterone (a male hormone). Females have much lower testosterone levels than males, but they secrete estrogen which enhances fat deposition in breasts and hips. Estrogen secretion does not increase muscle mass. When males combine strength training with their increased muscle mass, they can obtain greater upper and lower body strength than females. Moreover, strength is related not only to the muscle mass but also to the neuromuscular status and the ability to recruit more fibers by the nervous system. As we mentioned earlier, there are no gender differences in aerobic parameters. If the aerobic power parameter VO_2max is expressed per weight, both genders have similar values. However, because males have larger mass, the overall aerobic output is greater.

SKILLS

The acquisition of skills begins at birth and continues throughout life. Skills are dependent on the continued development of the neuromotor system. Skill also requires the coordination of the sense known as the perceptomotor system, which consists of the coordination of visual, kinesthetic, and auditory senses. Attainment of skills requires storage of learned information which depends on the continued repetition of the correct function. The development of the nervous system plays a critical role in skill development. At early stages of life, nerve myelination (insulation of the nerve from environment in order to conduct properly nerve impulses) is incomplete. This incomplete myelination results in slower nerve conduction and therefore less coordination than that of adults. At puberty both males and females experience a high rate of growth in height and weight, and development of neuromotor function.

Clumsiness is a fact of life with a pre-pubescent child. During this normal developmental period, the brain has to continuously adjust to the increased neuromotor function, as well as to the new spatial positions of the extremities (i.e., toes and fingers due to increased limb length). This hypothesis of the brain re-learning limb lengths can explain the clumsiness experienced during adolescence. There is data showing that males have a slight advantage in certain skills. However, more recent data on the same types of skills indicate that these differences are becoming smaller and smaller. This argues for social factors in skill levels of the two genders rather than inherent differences in the body physiology and biochemistry.

ATHLETIC AMENORRHEA

Athletic amenorrhea is the absence of the menstrual period for a length of time (e.g., greater than one year), and is associated with heavy exercise. Athletic amenorrhea is also strongly associated with the malfunction of the hypothalamus. The hypothalamus manufactures and secretes gonadotropin-releasing hormone (GnRH) in order to stimulate the pituitary gland which in turn releases follicle-stimulating hormone (FSH) and luteinizing hormone (LH). Both of these gonadotropins are involved in maintaining a normal menstrual cycle.

In the general population, the occurrence of amenorrhea averages about 5%; however, among heavy athletes it increases to 20 to 50%. For unknown reasons, ballet dancers, gymnasts, and runners have a higher incidence of athletic amenorrhea than other athletes. There is evidence that athletic amenorrhea is associated with the decrease in GnRH release from the hypothalamus. There are several factors that may contribute to athletic amenorrhea:

(1) Low body fat (below 17%). However, there are athletes with body fat well below 17% who have normal menstrual cycles

(2) Exercise may induce increased secretion of brain endorphins (natural morphine-like proteins in the body) such as opiates — which can inhibit GnRH secretion.

(3) Exercise may increase the secretion of melatonin from the brain. Melatonin can decrease GnRH secretion.

There are numerous factors contributing to athletic amenorrhea, and, more importantly, there is an interplay among these factors which contributes to the frequency of the disorder. The contributing factors include delayed puberty, stress (physical or emotional), poor nutrition (especially anorexia and bulimia), low body fat, heavy training (especially when combined with poor nutrition), genetic influence, and hormonal dysfunction. Amenorrhea can contribute to osteoporosis (decreased bone density), and the eventual loss of bone mass. Most symptoms of athletic amenorrhea are reversed when the factors contributing to amenorrhea cease to exist. However, there may not be a full recovery of bone mass. Therefore, if there is a delayed menarche (onset of menstrual cycle) or amenorrhea, the athlete should see her physician to determine which (if any) of these factors may be involved in her particular case.

Female athletes must monitor their iron levels. Due to menses, iron loss is large and if food intake is restricted, it could result in iron-deficiency. After consulting their physicians, the athlete may undergo iron supplementation. Equally, calcium levels in amenorrheic athlete maybe low. Special attention should be made to those athletes with repeat stress fractures. Calcium supplementation maybe prescribed by their physician.

FURTHER GENERAL READING

Colley & Beech (1988). Advances in Psychology. Cognition and Action in Skilled Behavior. Elsevier Science Publishers. pp. 273–331.

Haywood K. (1989). Life Span Motor Development. Human Kinetics Publishers, Inc.

Keogh et al. (1990). Movement Skill Development. Macmillian Publishing Company.

Whipp, B.J. and Ward, S.A. (1992). Will Women Soon Outrun Men? Nature 235:25.

Smyth & Wing (1984). The Psychology of Human Movement. Academic Press, Inc., pp. 215–240.

Glass A. et al. (1987). Amenorrhea in Olympic Marathon Runners. Fertility and Sterility 48:740–745

Henley K. et al. (1988). Exercise-Induced Menstrual Dysfunction. Ann. Rev. Med 39:443–451.

Jones K.P. et al. (1985). Comparison of Bone Density in Amenorrheic Woman Due to Athletics, Weight Loss, and Premature Menopause. Obstetrics and Gynecology 66:5–8.

Kaiserauer S. et al. (1988). Nutritional, Physiological, and Menstrual Status of Distance Runner. Med. and Sci. in Sports and Exer. 21:120–129.

Loucks A.B. et al. (1984). Exercise-Induced Stress Responses of Amenorrheic and Eumenorrheic Runners. J. of Clin. Endocrin. and Metab. 59:1109–1119.

White C.M. et al. (1990). Amenorrhea, Osteopenia, and the Female Athlete. Ped. Clinics of North Am. 37(5): 1125–1141.

Further General Reading

The following are the best general references for further reading. The reader can obtain a great deal more detailed knowledge from these books. However, they require some scientific background.

McArdle W.D. et al. (1991). Exercise Physiology. 3rd Edition, pp. 1–853. Lea & Febiger, Philadelphia (USA).

Wilmore J.H. et al. (1988). Training for Sport and Activity, 3rd edition, pp. 1–420, Wm. C. Brown Publishers, Dubuque, Iowa (USA).

American College of Sports Medicine (1991). Guidelines for Exercise Testing and Prescription, 4th edition, pp. 1–314. Lea and Febiger, Philadelphia (USA).

Committee on Sports Medicine and Fitness (1991). American Academy of Pediatrics, Sports Medicine: Health Care for Young Athlete. Second Edition American Academy of Pediatrics, Elk Grove Village, IL (USA).

Wolineky, I. and Hickson, Jr., J.F., Editors, (1994). "Nutrition in Exercise and Sport," 2nd edition, CRC Press, Boca Raton, Florida, pp. 1–416.

Malina, R.M. and Bouchard, C. (1991). Growth, Maturation and Physical Activity, pp. 1–463, Human Kinetics Books, Champaign, Illinois.

GLOSSARY

achilles tendon: the tendon joining the calf (gastronomius) and (soleus muscles) of the leg to the bone of the heel.

acromioclavicular joint: a joint located at the top of the shoulder formed by the scapula and clavicle.

adductor muscle: a muscle that draws towards the midline of the body.

Aerobic (exercise): when muscle contracts in the presence of oxygen.

amino acids: small organic compounds that are the building blocks for proteins. There are 20 amino acids.

amphetamines: a group of chemicals that stimulate the central nervous system. Often used as a street drug that is abused and can lead to psychosis, delusion, and in some cases, suicide. Street names for the drug are pep pills, speed, ice, black beauties, and lid poppers.

anaerobic (exercise): when muscle contracts in the absence of oxygen. For example, in sprinting the muscles function faster than the delivery system can provide sufficient oxygen. The breakdown of carbohydrates without oxygen causes the formation of lactic acid (lactate).

androgens: hormones that increase male characteristics.

analgesic: relieving pain (i.e., with the use of a drug).

anterior: toward the front frontal view, opposite to posterior.

anterior cruciate ligament: ligament that attaches the lateral side of the femur to the frontal side of the tibia

apophysis: projection from a bone.

arthrodesis: also called ankylosis. This is a surgical procedure to relieve pain or provide more support.

athletic amenorrhea: an irregular menstrual cycle often associated with heavy exercise.

ATP (Adenosine Triphosphate): An organic molecule used as the most prevalent energy currency in all cells of the body. It contains three phosphates linked together. The breakdown of the terminal phosphate releases energy utilized in numerous cellular functions. ATP is the source of energy for muscles.

autonomic nervous system: part of the nervous system that regulates involuntary body functions such as skeletal and cardiac muscles, smooth muscle (intestine) and glands. The system consists of two parts — the sympathetic nervous system in charge of increased heart rate, vasoconstriction and rise in blood pressure and the parasynpathetic nervous system in charge of slowing down heart rate, increases intestinal movement, and increases gland function.

avulsed: an injury involving torn skin.

ballistic stretching: the quick stretching of a muscle beyond its normal range. Not recommended.

blister: the formation of a fluid filled bubble which separates the skin from the underlying tissue.

blood pressure: the hydrostatic pressure exerted by circulating blood against the walls of arteries.

blood volume: the volume of the entire blood in the body — about 5 liters for a 70 kg person.

bone scan: the use of a radioactive substance injected into the vein along with an imaging device in order to visualize bone structure and possible pathology.

brace: a device which holds and supports any part of the body in the correct position while allowing it to function.

bronchospasm: constriction of the air passages in the tracheo-bronchial tree.

caffeine: a chemical compound found in coffee and chocolate. Caffeine is a central nervous system stimulant.

calcaneous: heel bone.

capillaries: small vessels that connect arteries and veins in tissues and muscles and allows the exchange of nutrients (e.g., oxygen, sugar) with waste products due to muscle activities.

carbohydrates: varied organic compounds such as saccharides and starches which serve as the main source of energy for the body. Gum and cellulose are also carbohydrates but humans lack the enzymes needed to digest them.

cardiovascular system: pertains to the heart and blood vessels. The heart pumps the blood into vessels to deliver nutrients to muscles and tissues and removes waste products.

cellulose: a specific kind of carbohydrate found in the cell walls of plants. The human body cannot digest cellulose.

cartilage: a tough elastic connective tissue found in joints, the end of bones, nose, and ears.

charlie horse: a sudden and painful cramping of the quadriceps or hamstring muscles. Usually due to the aggravation of damaged muscles by athletic activity.

compartment syndrome: an increased compression of the artery resulting in reduced blood flow. This is a serious pathology that could cause permanent damage to the hand or foot.

contusion: an injury to soft tissues without breakage in the skin.

cryotherapy: the use of cold temperature (i.e., ice) to lower metabolism in therapy of muscle injury.

dehydration: loss of water. Serious medical problem.

deltoid ligament: the medial ligament of the ankle joining medial malleolus with talus.

digitalis: an old drug that strengthens the heart pump.

displaced fracture: a fracture of a limb associated with deformity.

distal: away from

dorsiflex: upward movement to the back (i.e., when the foot moves towards the shin).

edema: excess fluid accumulation in tissue.

electrolytes: salts in solutions (i.e. body fluid) which dissociate into ions. For example, in such solution table salt dissociates into sodium ions (Na^+) and chloride ions (Cl^-). Body fluid electrolytes include Na^+, Cl^-, K^+, Mg^{2+}, Ca^{2+} and others. The maintenance of certain concentrations of electrolytes inside versus outside the cell is critical in maintaining the viability and function of the cell.

endorphine: chemical compounds (neuropeptides) secreted in the brain. Endorphines have many effects on the body; among them, feeling high, and analgesia. Endorphines are released during exercise.

endurance: ability of a person to perform a prolonged sporting event without adverse effects such as fatigue, exhaustion, or injury.

enzyme: a protein that catalyzes (speeds up) a reaction without being consumed.

epiphysis: the terminal end of a long bone.

ergogonic aids: any compound or activity that enhances the ability to achieve a greater work output.

exercise-induced asthma (EIB): a constriction of air passages in the tracheobronchial tree of the lungs experienced during exercise. Symptoms include: breathlessness, coughing, and wheezing.

extensor mechanism: the complex structure of muscles, ligaments, and tendons that stabilizes the patella and extends the knee.

fascia: an outer layer of fibrous connective tissue surrounding the muscle.

fats: a substance made up of lipids and fatty acids. Certain fats are important for body function. However, the intake of excess fats is associated with cardiovascular diseases.

femur: the bone in the thigh. It is the longest and biggest bone in the body.

fibrocartilaginous: composed of fibers and cartilages.

fibula: the smaller of the two bones of the leg just below the knee and above the ankle.

flat foot (pes planus): a common condition where the arch of the foot is flat.

follicle stimulating hormone (FSH): a hormone secreted by the brain that stimulates maturation of the follicle in the ovary and promotes the synthesis of sperms in males.

glucose: a simple sugar molecule found naturally in food such as fruits. It is the major source of energy in the cell.

glycogen: a compound made from glucose. It is the major form of stored energy in animal cells especially in the liver.

glycogen loading: the process by which an athlete loads his cells with excess glycogen by exercising heavily several days before the day of the event and eating large amounts of carbohydrates followed by rest the day before the event. This method stimulates the body to synthesize and store glycogen. In this manner, the athlete has a larger than normal amount of stored glycogen for utilization during the event.

glycolysis: an enzymatic process involving the breakdown of glycogen into simple sugars such as glucose. It is the sugars that are utilized to produce energy for the various cellular functions.

gonadotropin hormone: a hormone released by the brain that stimulates the function of testes and the ovaries.

gonadotropin releasing hormone: a hormone secreted by the brain that simulates the release of several hormones from the brain such as gonadotropin hormone, luteinizing hormone (LH) and follicle – stimulating hormone (FSH).

growth center: usually refers to the area at the end of the leg bones that increases in length during the growth period.

growth hormones: a hormone secreted by the brain that promotes all processes involved in growth and developments such as protein synthesis.

hamstring: a large muscle in the back of the thigh responsible for flexing the knee.

heat cramps: a muscle spasm associated with pain due to excess heat that results in loss of water and reduced blood flow to the muscle.

heat exhaustion: caused by depletion of the body of water. Symptoms include weakness and malaise.

heat stroke: prolonged exposure to heat and sun resulting in dehydration and loss of the thermal regulatory function. Symptoms include a sense of impending doom, headache, dizziness, confusion, and weakness. It is a serious medical emergency that could cause death.

heart rate: frequency of heart muscle contraction (beats) per minute.

heel spur: a bony projection at the back part of the foot — the calcaneus.

hematocrit: a measure of volume of packed cells in blood as percentage of blood volume. The normal range for men is 43%–49% and for women is 37%–43%.

hematoma: blood accumulation in damaged tissue.

hip pointer: damage to the attachments of the abdominal and thigh muscles to the back of the pelvis (iliac crest). A very painful injury.

hydrostatic pressure: amount of force exerted per unit surface area.

hyperinsulinemia: an excess amount of insulin secretion.

hypoglycemia: insufficient levels of sugar in the blood.

hypothalmus: a region in the brain involved in controlling body temperature, sleep, and appetite.

hypoxia: an insufficient concentration of oxygen in the tissue.

insulin: an important hormone secreted by the pancreas involved in the enhancement of energy storage in the cell such as the removal of glucose from the blood into the cell and forming glycogen from glucose.

intermetatarsal: in between the metatarsal bones of the foot.

ischemia: reduced oxygenated blood flow to the tissue.

isokinetic: a special method of exercise where tension develops as the muscle contracts.

isotonic: muscle contraction with constant resistance.

krebs cycle: a sequence of biochemical reactions that breakdown sugars, fatty acids, and amino acids into carbon dioxide and water. The krebs cycle produces ATP (Adenosine Triphosphate) — the energy currency for the body.

lactate (lactic acid): an organic acid produced when muscles perform work in the absence of oxygen (an anaerobic process).

lactate shift: a shift to a higher level of tolerance of the blood lactate level due to endurance training.

ligament: fibrous tissue that connects bones to bones. It is present in joints for strength and stability.

luteinizing hormone (LH): a hormone secreted by the brain that stimulates the secretion of sex hormones in the ovary and testes.

macrotrauma: destruction of large and visible amounts of tissue due to inappropriate or accidental use of a tissue.

medial: toward the midline.

melatonin: a hormone secreted by the brain (the only hormone produced by the pineal gland) that is involved in gondotropic hormones, skin pigmentation, and many other important functions.

metabolism: refers to all biochemical processes in the body that are involved in areas such as growth, development, energy production, and repair.

metatarsal: bones of the foot.

microcirculation: refers to the blood flow of smaller blood vessels such as capillaries. This system allows for the exchange of oxygen from blood to the tissues and the removal of waste products of exercise such as carbon dioxide and lactate from the tissue.

microtrauma: destruction of a few cells at a time due to a repetitive movement.

mitochondria: an organelle in the cell specializing in the production of ATP (Adenosine Triphosphate).

motor unit: the smallest functional muscle fiber within a motor neuron.

muscle: specialized elongated cells that have the capability to contract and relax, thus causing movement.

muscle fibers (Type I, II): the component of muscle. Muscle fibers are formed by a collection of muscle cells and can specialize either in long lasting endurance, a burst of contractions or medium activity. Type I refers to the long lasting fibers used in marathon running. Type IIA are defined as the sprint type fibers and Type IIB is in between Type IIB and Type I.

myelination: a sheath of tissue surrounding the nerves acting as an electrical insulator.

myoglobin: carrier of oxygen in muscle. A counterpart to hemoglobin as the oxygen carrier in the blood.

navicular: refers to a boat shape. Usually, navicular bones refer to boat shaped bones in the foot and hand.

oblique: somewhere between horizontal and perpendicular.

Osgood Schlatter Disease: when the patellar tendon insertion into the tibia is pulled forcefully causing a tibial nodule. This disease is found mainly in adolescence and is associated with pain and swelling of the knee.

ossification: the formation of bone (mostly calcium deposits called calcification).

osteochondritis dissecans: bone fragment separation in a joint.

osteoporosis: loss of bone density usually associated with older women.

overload principle: a gradual increase in workload which results in greater endurance, power, and muscle size.

oxidation: the breakdown of chemicals involving oxygen (oxygen receives an electron from hydrogen). Usually this process occurs in the mitochondria, the power house of the cell.

patella: kneecap.

peritendinitis: inflammation of the tendon sheet usually accompanied with pain and swelling.

pH: the negative logarithm of hydrogen ion concentration (i.e. a measure of hydrogen ion concentration). A pH value of 7.0 is neutral, above 7.0 is alkaline, and below 7.0 is acidic.

phalange: bones of the finger or toes.

phosphocreatine phosphate: a small organic compound with high energy that can quickly form adenosine triphosphate (ATP) as a source of energy when needed without going through aerobic or anaerobic systems.

phosphorylation: the addition of phosphate onto a compound.

planta fascia: fibrous tissue that supports the bottom of the foot.

plasma: the straw-colored fluid portion of the blood consisting of water, electrolytes, proteins, glucose, and others (i.e., the liquid portion of the blood).

plica: folding of the tissue.

posterior: view from the back, opposite to anterior.

progressive principle: increasing overload gradually in order to avoid fatigue and injury.

proprioception: ability to sense body parts positions in space.

protein: a large naturally occurring compound consisting of many amino acids. Proteins are involved in most cellular functions such as enzymes, structure, antibodies, ... etc.

puberty: period of life when males and females become capable of reproduction.

quadriceps (muscle): the four components of muscle at the front of the thigh — vastus medialis, vastus lateralis, vastus intermedius, and rectus emoris.

respiratory system: breathing system.

sacrum: the back bone area of the pelvis.

serum: the remaining liquid after blood clots. When blood clots, it separate the solid components such as blood cells, platelets, and clotting factors from the remaining fluid called serum.

shin splint: tendenitis (inflammation) of the tibial area of the leg.

shock: collapse and sudden inability of the cardiovascular system to provide enough blood circulation to the body.

specificity principle: a training model that emphasizes that training must resemble the sporting activity for which the athlete is training.

splint: a mechanical device used to immobilize a part of the body.

sprain: injury to a ligament.

starch: the main storage food in plants. It consist of long chains of glucose molecules. The counterpart to starch in animals is glycogen.

static stretching: stretching the muscle to a position of slight discomfort and holding it at that position for a period of time.

steroids: chemicals share common structure with the steroid hormones.

steroid hormones: natural hormones in the body such as androgens and estrogens involved in sex characteristics and other important functions.

strain: overstretching or tearing of a muscle or a tendon.

stress fracture: when a bone is subjected to repeated and frequent stress, like running on a hard pavement, it causes microfracture of the bone associated with low level of pain.

stroke volume: blood volume ejected per heart beat.

subluxation: partial dislocation.

subscapularis: one of the shoulder bones of the rotator cuff.

synovial (fluid): lubricating fluid in the joints.

talus: ankle bone.

tarsal bones: bones (seven of them) at the back of the foot.

tendon: fibrous tough tissue that attaches skeletal muscle to bones.

tendinitis: inflammation of the tendon which, in the context of sports is due to injury.

thermoregulatory system: a structure located in the hypothalamus responsible for the regulation of normal body temperature.

tibia: shin bone (the largest of the two adjacent leg bones).

triglycerides: a type of fat consisting of a fatty acid and a compound called glycerol.

turf toe: a sprain of the joint (metatarsophalangeal) of the large toe.

vasoconstriction: narrowing of the blood vessels.

vasodilation: expansion of the blood vessels.

viscosity: a parameter of fluid characteristics that relates to the ability of fluid solution to flow easily.

VO$_2$max: maximal oxygen uptake by the person due to increased level of exercise.

Index

A

Abdominal exercises 33
Active rest 22
Adaptation 92–97
Adenosine Triphosphate (ATP) 18
Adolescents 3
Aerobic 23
Amenorrhea 118
Amphetamine 12
Anaerobic 11, 12
Ankle 55
Anterior cruciate ligament (ACL) 60

B

Back exercises 33
Blisters 50
Blood sugar 102
Body composition 4, 15
Body fat 119

C

Caffeine 112
Calcium 97
Carbohydrates 8, 102, 103, 106
Cardiovascular 23
Circuit training 25
Clicking 76
Compartment syndrome 56
Compression 49
Conditioning 5
Contusions 46, 64
Coordination 4
Cryotherapy 47

D

Deadarm 69
Dehydration 83
Discipline 4
Drugs 109

E

Elbow
    injuries 74
Electrolytes 85
Elevation 49
Endurance 4, 12, 13, 92
    cardiorespiratory 92, 93
    cardiovascular 23
Energy 16, 104
    stored 104
    pyramid 19
Exercise Induced Asthma (EIA) 79
Extensor mechanism 60

F

Fatigue 19
Fats 8, 106

Fiber composition   95
Fielders progression   39
Fitness   4
Fitness evaluation   13
Flat foot   52
Flexibility   4, 14
   exercises   6
   program   28
Fluid loss   82
Foot   51
Forearm exercises   32

G

Glycogen   18, 104
Glycolysis   11, 18
Growth Hormone (GH)   111
Growth spurt   3

H

Hand injuries   77
Head injuries   78
Heart rate   23
Heat cramps   86
Heat exhaustion   86
Heat stroke   87
Heavy training   9
Hip   65
Hyperinsulenemia   9
Hypoglycemia   9

I

Interval training   25
Isotonic   14

K

Knee   58
Kneecap   60

L

Lactate   19, 94
Leg   56
Little league pitchers   39
Lower extremities injuries   50
Lower extremity program   34

M

Management of injuries   41, 42, 44
Minerals   8
Motivation   4
Muscle   5, 60, 63, 117
   protein   10
   soreness   5
Myoglobin   95

N

Neck injuries   78
Nutrition   7, 102

O

Osgood schlatters   61
Osteochondritis dissecans   62
Overload   21
Oxidation   18

P

Phosphocreatine phosphate (PCr)   18
Pitcher's shoulder program   30
Plantar fasciitis   52
Plica syndrome   62
Popping   76
Power   14
Practice sessions   5
Pre-game meals   9
Proprioception   15
Proteins   8, 105
   sparing   103
Puberty   3

Q

Quadriceps   60

R

Range of Motion (ROM)   72
RICE   47
Running program   27

S

Severe's apophysitis   52
Shin splints   57
Shoulder injuries   74
Shoulder strengthening for pitchers   29
Skills   5, 118
Skin fold   16
Sport drinks   85
Sprains   46, 55
Steroids   110
Strength   21, 24
Stress   5
Stress fracture   54, 56
Stretching static   20
Sweating   82

T

Tendon   61
Thigh   63
Time to peak endurance   6
Training   21
   active rest   11
   frequency   6, 22
   intensity   6
   overload   11
   progressive   11, 22
Turf toe   50

U

Upper body exercises   31
Upper extremity injuries   65

V

Vitamins   8, 106

W

Water   8, 82
Wrist   77, 78

1740